MEDICAL DEVICES AND EQUIPMENT

CREATING 21ST CENTURY MEDICAL DEVICES: DEVELOPMENT NEEDS AND ISSUES

MEDICAL DEVICES AND EQUIPMENT

Additional books in this series can be found on Nova's website at:

https://www.novapublishers.com/catalog/index.php?cPath=23_29&seriesp=Medical+Devices+and+Equipment

Additional E-books in this series can be found on Nova's website at:

https://www.novapublishers.com/catalog/index.php?cPath=23_29&seriespe=Medical+Devices+and+Equipment

MEDICAL DEVICES AND EQUIPMENT

CREATING 21ST CENTURY MEDICAL DEVICES: DEVELOPMENT NEEDS AND ISSUES

NELSON E. PARKER
EDITOR

Nova
Nova Science Publishers, Inc.
New York

LIBRARY OF CONGRESS CATALOGING-IN-PUBLICATION DATA

ISBN: 978-1-60876-773-1

Available Upon Request

Published by Nova Science Publishers, Inc. † New York

CONTENTS

PREFACE

In order to be legally manufactured in the U.S., medical devices must be approved by the Food and Drug Administration (FDA), the agency responsible for protecting the public health by assuring the safety, efficacy, and security of human medical devices and other products. The regulation of medical devices can affect their cost, quality, and availability in the health care system. This book discusses the legislative history of medical device regulation, describes the FDA's approval process for medical devices, and provides an overview of the medical device related legislative issues facing Congress.

Chapter 1 - This government report presents the perspectives of the senior scientists of the NITRD Program's High Confidence Software and Systems (HCSS) Coordinating Group (CG), with input from experts from other Federal agencies, on the R&D challenges, needs, and strategies for developing and deploying the next generations of high-confidence[1] medical devices, software, and systems. HCSS agencies whose missions are not medical device-specific have found it beneficial to partner in this area because medical device research challenges are similar, if not identical, to those within their purview.

Digital technologies are increasingly being assigned high-level control over the monitoring, sensing, actuation, and communications of medical devices – often with human life in the balance. Through this report and associated HCSS-sponsored national workshops, the HCSS agencies are seeking to illuminate fundamental scientific and technical challenges that must be addressed before we can design and build high-confidence devices, software, and systems that operate flawlessly from end to end.

The report seeks to paint the landscape of the evolution of medical device technology and the Federal investments that have benefitted medical device R&D over time. Future R&D needs and strategies are discussed in the context of this landscape.

Chapter 2 - The Food and Drug Administration (FDA) within the Department of Health and Human Services (HHS) is responsible for oversight of medical devices sold in the United States. Regulations place devices into three classes, with class III including those with the greatest risk to patients. Unless exempt by regulation, new devices must clear FDA premarket review via either the 510(k) premarket notification process, which determines if a new device is substantially equivalent to another legally marketed device, or the more stringent premarket approval (PMA) process, which requires the manufacturer to supply evidence providing reasonable assurance that the device is safe and effective. Class III devices must generally obtain an approved PMA, but until FDA issues regulations requiring submission of PMAs, certain types of class III devices may be cleared via the 510(k) process. The FDA

Amendments Act of 2007 mandated that GAO study the 510(k) process. GAO examined which premarket review process—510(k) or PMA—FDA used to review selected types of device submissions in fiscal years 2003 through 2007. GAO reviewed FDA data and regulations, and interviewed FDA officials.

Chapter 3 - The Food and Drug Administration (FDA) is the agency responsible for ensuring the safety and effectiveness of medical devices. An establishment may not market a device in the United States without FDA's prior approval or clearance.

In 2002, Congress first granted FDA the authority to collect user fees from medical device establishments. The authority was granted to help reduce the time required for the agency to review and make decisions about marketing applications. Lengthy review times harmed establishments, which waited to market devices, and patients, who waited to use them. User fee law provides a revenue stream for the agency, and also requires it to set *performance goals* for rapid application review.

The authority to collect medical device user fees has been authorized in five-year increments, and will expire next on October 1, 2012. In 2002, it was first established in the Medical Device User Fee and Modernization Act (MDUFMA; P.L. 107-250). Before reauthorization, it was amended by the Medical Device Technical Corrections Act (P.L. 108-214) and the Medical Device User Fee Stabilization Act of 2005 (P.L. 109-43). It has been reauthorized once, in the Medical Device User Fee Amendments of 2007 (MDUFA 2007), enacted as Title II of the Food and Drug Administration Amendments Act of 2007 (H.R. 3580; P.L. 110-85).

Since medical device user fees were first collected in FY2003, they have comprised an increasing proportion of FDA's device budget. In FY2003, $14.8 million of user fees comprised 6.8% of the budget. In FY2007 (the year of the most recent reauthorization), $35.2 million of user fees comprised 13.2% of the budget.

Medical device user fees have raised a number of issues. These have prompted Congress to determine the following: which activities should require fees; how user fees can be kept from supplanting federal funding, or being diverted from device review (through *triggers*); which activities the agency should fund with user fees; and how to qualify as a small business. (Small businesses pay reduced fee amounts.)

In addition to addressing the above issues, medical device user fee legislation has served a secondary purpose as a moving vehicle that legislators could use to address a range of issues related to medical devices. For example, MDUFA 2007 included provisions about the extent to which FDA can delegate activities to third parties (inspections and the review of premarket notifications); establishment registration requirements (timing and electronic submission); a unique device identification system; reporting requirements for devices linked to serious injuries or deaths; and requirements that FDA and GAO conduct certain studies. MDUFMA included provisions about reprocessed single use devices and other topics.

This report provides an overview of FDA and the medical device review process. It then presents the legislative history of user fees. Next, it explains the basics of FDA's medical device user fee system, noting the way in which various provisions have evolved. Finally, it provides an overview of non-user fee issues addressed in the device user fee acts. This report will be updated as events warrant.

Chapter 4 - The central medical device issue for Congress is how best to help speed medical devices to consumers if they are safe and effective, and correct them or keep them from consumers if they are not. A medical device may be anything from a tongue depressor to a pacemaker. In order to be legally marketed in the United States, medical devices must be approved by the Food and Drug Administration (FDA), the agency responsible for protecting the public health by assuring the safety, efficacy, and security of human medical devices and other products. FDA's Center for Devices and Radiological Health (CDRH) is primarily responsible for medical device review. The regulation of medical devices can affect their cost, quality, and availability in the health care system.

During reviews, FDA classifies devices according to the risk they pose to consumers. If a premarket review is warranted by the potential risk, a manufacturer must demonstrate that its device is safe and effective, or substantially equivalent to a device already on the market. FDA requires product manufacturers to register their facilities, list their devices with FDA, and follow general controls requirements. Manufacturers of FDA-approved devices are required to report serious adverse events associated with the use of their devices to FDA. In addition, tracking is required for some medical devices.

The medical device approval process is currently funded through direct FDA appropriations from Congress, and increasingly through user fees collected from applicants. FDA's authority to collect user fees, originally authorized in 2002 (P.L. 107-250), has been reauthorized in five-year increments. It will next expire on October 1, 2012, under the terms of the FDA Amendments Act of 2007 (P.L. 110-85).

A number of medical device related topics are of interest to members of the 111th Congress. These include liability and preemption, the 501(k) clearance process, Medicare and other federal coverage, importation and inspection, advertising, the regulation of *in vitro* diagnostic products (IVDs, which are laboratory tests), and some other issues.

This report contains the legislative history of medical device regulation, describes FDA's approval process for medical devices, and provides an overview of the medical device related legislative issues facing Congress.

In: Creating 21st Century Medical Devices
Editor: Nelson E. Parker

ISBN: 978-1-60876-773-1

Chapter 1

HIGH-CONFIDENCE MEDICAL DEVICES: CYBER-PHYSICAL SYSTEMS FOR 21ST CENTURY HEALTH CARE*

Networking and Information Technology Research and Development Program

ABOUT THIS REPORT AND THE HCSS NATIONAL WORKSHOP SERIES

This government report presents the perspectives of the senior scientists of the NITRD Program's High Confidence Software and Systems (HCSS) Coordinating Group (CG), with input from experts from other Federal agencies, on the R&D challenges, needs, and strategies for developing and deploying the next generations of high-confidence[1] medical devices, software, and systems. HCSS agencies whose missions are not medical device-specific have found it beneficial to partner in this area because medical device research challenges are similar, if not identical, to those within their purview.

Digital technologies are increasingly being assigned high-level control over the monitoring, sensing, actuation, and communications of medical devices – often with human life in the balance. Through this report and associated HCSS-sponsored national workshops, the HCSS agencies are seeking to illuminate fundamental scientific and technical challenges that must be addressed before we can design and build high-confidence devices, software, and systems that operate flawlessly from end to end.

The report seeks to paint the landscape of the evolution of medical device technology and the Federal investments that have benefitted medical device R&D over time. Future R&D needs and strategies are discussed in the context of this landscape.

The government authors provide analytical commentary on findings and recommendations made in a 2006 workshop report produced by academic and industry scientists from an HCSS-sponsored planning meeting held in November 2004 and a follow-

---

* This is an edited, reformatted and augmented version of a Networking and Information Technology Research and Development Program publication dated February 2009.

on National Workshop on High Confidence Medical Devices, Software, and Systems (HCMDSS) held in June 2005. (See Appendix 3 for the workshop participants' report.) The agency perspectives also address issues that arose from an HCSS-co-sponsored workshop in 2007 on High Confidence Medical Devices, Software, and Systems and Medical Device Plug-and-Play Interoperability held in cooperation with the University of Pennsylvania, the Center for the Integration of Medicine and Innovative Technology (CIMIT), the Massachusetts General Hospital, and Partners Healthcare. Federal sponsors include the Agency for Healthcare Research and Quality (AHRQ), the Food and Drug Administration (FDA), the National Institute of Standards and Technology (NIST), the National Security Agency (NSA), the National Science Foundation (NSF), and the U.S. Army Telemedicine and Advanced Technology Research Center (TATRC) [3], along with the National Coordination Office for NITRD (NCO/NITRD). This report also draws from *Software for Dependable Systems: Sufficient Evidence?,* a 2007 National Academies study that was commissioned by HCSS agencies in 2003.

The medical device workshops had three main goals: 1) *to provide a forum* for leaders and visionaries from industry, research laboratories, academia, and the Federal government to identify crucial challenges facing the current design, manufacture, certification, and use of high-confidence medical devices, software, and systems; 2) *to identify promising research directions* that could revolutionize the way medical technologies are designed, built, and validated, so that high confidence could be designed into devices, software, and systems right from the start; and 3) *to grow a sustainable multidisciplinary research and development community* for the advancement of high-confidence medical devices, software, and systems.

More than 100 experts participated in each of the larger workshops. The participants represented a broad mix of the relevant stakeholders – including medical researchers, device developers, Federal government regulators, and users (both medical practitioners and caregivers) – with expertise in medicine, technology, and assurance. The workshop participants' report offers their conclusions about research priorities that should be addressed over identified timeframes. The conclusions of the participants' report are those of its authors and do not necessarily represent the position of the NITRD Program or its member agencies.

These workshops are part of a broader series of national workshops undertaken by the HCSS group to identify the research needed to enable the design, manufacture, and certification of future high-confidence software and systems in multiple life-, safety-, security-, and missioncritical domains of strategic interest to the Nation. To date, these workshops have focused on five domain areas: 1) high-confidence medical devices, software, and systems; 2) supervisory control and data acquisition (SCADA) systems and digital control systems (DCS); 3) aviation systems certification; 4) next-generation platforms and technologies for cyber-physical systems, and 5) high-confidence automotive and transportation cyber-physical systems. Future reports will focus on manufacturing, net zero-energy buildings, and power generation.

EXECUTIVE SUMMARY

Overview

The U.S. market for medical devices[3] is the largest in the world. At an estimated $83 billion in 2006, this market represents nearly half the global total and is growing at 6 percent annually – about double the rate of U.S. GDP.[4]

With the advent of microprocessors, miniaturization of electronic circuits, wired and wireless digital networking, and new materials and manufacturing processes, older generations of mechanical and analog electromechanical devices used in patient diagnosis, monitoring, and treatment have largely been replaced by devices and systems based on information technologies across the diverse array of contemporary medical devices. They are often connected to other devices in increasingly complex configurations, potentially creating systems of systems that span scales from tiny (e.g., an ingestible digital camera with real-time video) to ultra-large (e.g., scanning and irradiation equipment and geographically distributed electronic records systems).

The emerging classes of IT-enabled medical devices mark a significant paradigm shift: What used to be essentially passive devices controlled by a human operator are now complex computing systems whose embedded sensors and actuators not only monitor, *but actively control,* critical physiological processes and functions. The embedded computing, sensing, modeling, communications, and deep integration with physical elements and processes allows these new "cyber-physical systems" to achieve levels of functionality, adaptability, and effectiveness not possible with simpler passive systems.

Government Perspectives

The authors of this report, senior scientists of the NITRD Program's High Confidence Software and Systems (HCSS) Coordinating Group (CG), point to fundamental scientific and technical challenges posed by the rapidly expanding digital environment in medicine and health care. They identify critical research advances that are needed to enable the design and manufacture of new generations of increasingly complex, interconnected, and interoperating medical device cyberphysical systems that will offer innovative new capabilities and function far more safely, securely, and reliably than today's medical devices. The authors believe that the key findings and conclusions, while directed at medical devices, relate strongly to other domains of interest to NITRD organizations.

Key Findings

> Today's medical device architectures are typically proprietary, not interoperable, and rely on professionals to provide inputs and assess outputs; "families" of such devices also tend to be stove-piped and not interoperable with other "families" of devices.
> In the frequent circumstance that a patient is connected to multiple devices at once, such as in an operating room, clinicians now must monitor all devices independently, synthesize data, and act on their observations, which can be affected by stress, fatigue, or other human factors.

Medical device architecture is beginning to include wired and wireless interfaces to facilitate networked communication of patient data. But ad hoc efforts to aggregate data across devices designed to operate separately can lead to unintended or accidental results.

The growing interest in such capabilities as home health care services, delivery of expert medical practice remotely (telemedicine), and online clinical lab analysis underscores the central role of advanced networking and distributed communication of medical information in the health systems of the future. Increased R&D focus on the specialized engineering of networked medical device systems is needed.

Neither past nor current development methods are adequate for the high-confidence design and manufacture of highly complex, interoperable medical device software and systems ("intelligent" prosthetics, minimally invasive surgical devices, implants, "operating room of the future"), which in years to come will likely include nano/bio devices, bionics, or even pure (programmable) biological systems.

Today's verification and validation (V&V) efforts are driven by system-life-cycle-development activities that rely primarily on methods of post-hoc inspection and testing; these approaches are inadequate in the face of the diversity and complexity of components and interactions in emerging medical devices and systems.

Today, scientific principles and engineering foundations are lacking that could enable both the design and assurance of high-confidence medical device cyber-physical systems.

Conclusions

Clearly, there is a need for rationally designed high-confidence medical device cyber-physical architectures; a strategic focus on R&D in compositional modeling and design is needed to address the open systems needs, respond to technological innovation, and bridge the jointly cyber and physical aspects of this complex systems problem.

An open research community of academics and medical device manufacturers is needed to create strategies for development of end-to-end, principled, engineering-based design and development tools. Certifying component devices is necessary, but not sufficient; a key area of research needed is the incremental certified composition of certified components.

Manufacturers will need access to open, formally composable V&V technology that relies on computational models unifying cyber and physical systems to help establish sufficient evidence. A key V&V research challenge is to understand what is meant by the term "sufficient evidence,"[5] its properties, and how this can be accepted in the global economy.

The HCSS group recommends that a strategic R&D focus on high-confidence networking and IT for the design, implementation, and certification of **open medical technologies** be undertaken, both to meet the goals of cost-effective, improved patient care and to spur innovation that promotes U.S. leadership in biomedical technology.

To enable the necessary holistic cyber-physical systems understanding, barriers must fall among the relevant disciplines: medicine, discrete and continuous mathematics

of dynamics and control; real-time computation and communication; medical robotics; learning; computational models and the supporting systems engineering design, analysis, and implementation technologies; and formal and algorithmic methods for stating, checking, and reasoning about system properties.
Incentives are needed to enable effective cooperation between government, industry, and academia to build the underpinning standards and networking and information technology frameworks (e.g., testbeds) for developing open, interoperable medical cyber-physical systems.

THE EVOLUTION OF MEDICAL DEVICES

The U.S. market for medical devices is the largest in the world. At an estimated $83 billion in 2006, it constitutes nearly half the global total. This market accounts for approximately 4.1 percent of total U.S. health-care expenditures, and it is growing at approximately 6 percent per year – about double the rate of U.S. GDP.[6] The industry is highly diversified, ranging from single individuals working out of their homes to global conglomerates. In the United States, the industry is one the most high-end employers by salary, with more than 350,000 workers in 2006. Of the approximately 8,500 U.S. medical device firms, over 80 percent have fewer than 50 employees.[7] The medical devices produced by this industry are similarly diverse, ranging from digital thermometers to prosthetics, cochlear implants to proton beam therapy systems, and hospital health care systems.

Past, Present, and Emerging Medical Device Systems

As in many industries, the technology in medical devices has evolved in tandem with overall technology innovation and the establishment of engineering best practices, transitioning from vacuum tube electronics to transistor-based electronics and from metal to plastics. Prior to the digital age, medical devices were generally built using analog components in relatively simple designs, with relatively simple user interfaces and limited functionality. The primary method of controlling risk to patients was competent human intervention. Life spans of these devices tended to be rather long, corresponding to the rate of technological change and established business models.

Over the last 20 or so years, designs for medical devices have evolved from analog to digital systems. Today, software, microprocessor, sensor, and actuator technologies are ubiquitous in these devices. Some of the more complex devices can have a million lines or more of code. Most devices contain *embedded systems* that rely on a combination of proprietary, commercial-off-the-shelf (COTS) and custom software or software-of-unknown-pedigree (SOUP) components. These systems are highly proprietary and increasingly dependent on software to provide greater levels of device robustness and functionality. Designs continue to rely, however, on competent human intervention as the ultimate risk-control measure.

An *embedded system* may be thought of as a special-purpose computer system often designed to perform dedicated functions and subject to resource-limitation constraints as part of a mechanical device. Often embedded system programs are implemented in read-only memory and are not intended to be generally reprogrammable. (In contrast, general-purpose computing systems, such as PCs, execute a wide variety of functions and are easily reprogrammed.) Embedded systems are becoming critical in medicine because they increasingly *control* functions of, and communicate with, patients themselves as well as engineered systems. Device life spans are shrinking due to more rapid innovation in enabling technologies and the demand for more robust systems. The pressures of rising health care costs, an aging population[8], and diminishing medical professional resources are also driving health-care providers to seek technological innovations to maintain or improve patient care as efficiently as possible.

Issues in Current Medical Device Systems

Architectures

Device architectures are highly proprietary, not interoperable, and rely heavily on professionals to provide inputs and assess outputs. Embedded systems are, for the most part, open-loop[9]. Exceptions (closed-loop) tend to be implantable devices such as implantable cardioverter defibrillators (ICDs) or cochlear prosthetics (with soft operational deadlines). Any network communication is largely for the purpose of diagnostic output. Complex instruction set computer (CISC) and reduced instruction set computer (RISC) architectures are commonly used. Multicore and system-on-a-chip (SoC) architectures and flexible reconfigurable architectures, such as field programmable gate arrays (FPGAs), are becoming more common in device designs.

Development Methods

Current software development methods range from older methods such as structured programming to object-oriented programming paradigms where objects are instantiated at run-time. Formal methods-based design and analysis are not widely used. Human resource-intensive, system-based verification and validation activities are conducted to demonstrate that a device will perform as intended. Use of static-analysis tools on implemented code is limited. Development platforms do not facilitate integration of hardware, software, and human factors in design, development, and manufacturing.

Research Challenges

- *Platform and implementation technologies are needed that support science- and engineering-based design, development, and certification.*
- *An open research community needs to be established comprising academics and medical device manufacturers to create strategies for the development of end-to-end, principled, engineering-based design and development tools.*
    - Strengths and properties of tools should be easily understood, inherently trustable, and scalable so they can be applied appropriately to the particular task.
    - Tools and the science behind them should be interoperable and complementary.
    - Their results must be trustable relative to some national or international standard to facilitate certification.

- *Additional research is needed to reduce the number of false positives and negatives in commercially available static analyzers.*
- *Formal methods-based design techniques must scale to human resource-intensive processes.* An example is modeling work-flow practices of providers or caregivers.

In addition to addressing these research challenges, it is important to ensure that a credible "faster, better, cheaper" business case can be made to persuade device manufacturers to change their design and development practices and open markets to new participation.

Issues in Emerging Medical Device Systems

Emerging medical device systems may be characterized as those systems that are pushing the envelope of regulated technology. Examples are closed-loop or networked device systems.

In today's health care environment, it is common to have a patient connected to several medical devices simultaneously. These devices may be delivering drugs, regulating breathing, or reporting a physiological status. Caregivers must aggregate, analyze, and react to this information in a coordinated way. In the operating room, for example, one may find many devices providing life-supporting functions and multiple medical professionals *interoperating* based on information provided by the various devices (and their own observations). Humans are subject to fatigue, miscommunication, distractions, misinterpretation of information, information overload, and other factors. These factors can combine to contribute to an undesirable patient outcome.

The digital technology found in most medical devices today would make it rather easy (at least conceptually) to collect device information, aggregate it, and either present it to a health care provider for some action or use it to trigger an autonomous action by a device. For example, it is routine to simultaneously display data from pulse oximeters, EKGs, and blood-pressure devices to monitor patients with cardiac problems; devices delivering radiation treatment to a tumor in an organ that moves can sense organ motion and direct a radiation beam calibrated to the movement.

The need to provide health care services in a home care environment, or deliver expert medical practice remotely (telemedicine, emergency response), or perform online clinical lab analysis further underscores the central role of advanced networking and distributed communication of medical information (via electronic health records) in emerging care systems. Adding computing and control mechanisms to the critical medical information communicated (via networking) establishes a fundamental prerequisite to high-confidence cyber-physical medical systems. This must be done in a way that supports the principled development and implementation of systems of medical systems.

Architectures

Emerging medical device architecture is beginning to provide wired and wireless interfaces to facilitate networked communication of device (patient) data. But as the workshop participants' report suggests, attempts to aggregate medical data between devices that were designed to operate separately are resulting in unintended or accidental (virtual) couplings.

The device procurement process historically has established "stove-piped families" of proprietary devices that are not designed to interoperate with other "families" of devices. Ad-hoc attempts to integrate provider processes and the families of proprietary devices have resulted in very loosely coupled "stealth" networks that can involve transferring data between devices via memory stick, PDA (Bluetooth and IR communication), barcoding, or other technologies.

Clearly, there is a need for rationally designed high-confidence medical device cyber-physical architectures.

To optimize patient care, multiple cyber-physical devices must interoperate together smoothly at a very high level of confidence. Interoperability facilitates and accelerates aggregation of patient information that can be used to improve patient care and treatment outcomes. To that end, we see emerging efforts of health care providers to develop closed-loop interoperable medical systems. The workshop participants' report describes some of the issues involved.

Development Methods

Neither past nor current development methods are adequate for engineering these complex emerging medical systems. As mentioned in the workshop participants' report, there is a need to be able reliably to compose, not only highly trustworthy systems from diverse components, but also highly trustworthy systems of systems. Medical device design oriented toward a holistic approach that integrates functional, computational, and communication designs in the presence of uncertain patient models in both normal and abnormal conditions is needed.

It is our view that the emerging development methods must scale across the device industry's entire problem set as well as its diverse development skill levels. The ability for third parties to trust all aspects of design and development results is key to device innovation.

Research Challenges

The workshop participants' report identifies a number of important areas for next steps in research for laying the foundation for high-confidence cyber-physical medical devices and systems. Additional areas for consideration are:

> *Synthesizing medical information.* As medical systems evolve into cyber-physical systems, the notions of feedback and interoperability will most likely emulate the practice of medicine itself. This presents significant challenges in encapsulating medical information because different doctors may envision varying treatment regimes for a given patient and doctors in diverse specializations approach medical information differently.

QoS guarantees. Advances are needed in networked embedded-control systems technology so that QoS guarantees at the component level also guarantee performance at the system level. The relative importance of security, privacy, robustness, interoperability, extensibility, and mobility, as well as general patient safety, must be evaluated carefully.

Dynamic management of large-scale systems. The workshop participants' report touched on the notion of dynamic medical-system configurability in the context of plug-and-play (PnP) systems. However, the bounds of the PnP system were not explicitly characterized. One could imagine the system being implemented by a diversity of providers at the local, state, and national (perhaps even international) levels. Managing resources and configurations (including device versions, legacy systems, etc.) implemented in such a varied landscape is truly a grand challenge.

Trust in abstractions. The workshop participants' report identifies the need for more robust means of modeling and formal methods-based checking and verification of medical-device designs. In a more general sense, virtually every step of a development process is based on some level of system abstraction or composition of abstractions. Research is needed to provide a scalable means of being able to trust abstractions and their properties, and their interfaces to other abstractions and concrete equivalents.

The security challenge. While the workshop report identifies medical-device system security as a research challenge, further emphasis is needed to comprehend the full scope of the issue. The notion of medical device system security is in its infancy. This is because, in general, most medical devices are not connected to a network. However, as noted above, this architectural paradigm is changing. As health care records evolve from paper to electronic media and as this information is used pervasively in medical device interoperation, security issues are going to become critical.

Future Medical Devices: High-Confidence Cyber-Physical Systems (CPS)

As technological advances and innovation permit medical device systems to decrease in size while increasing in capabilities, it is reasonable to expect that future devices could evolve into ubiquitous supervisory-control, patient-centric systems performing autonomous, cooperative, and coordinated actions.

Architectures

Ongoing research seems headed toward the merging of physiological, biological, engineered, and physical systems for health care that include, for example, biomechanical systems, nano/bio devices, bionics, or even pure (programmable) biological systems. Enabled by advances in both biological understanding and IT, medical devices and systems of the future can be expected to continue the trend towards heterogeneous configurable personalized systems far more capable, and also more complex, than today's.

Development Methods

As the architecture of medical systems evolves from the domain of macro- and micro-mechanical systems to nanoscale CPS and biological systems, development methods must fundamentally change. It is likely that a greater dependence on, and trust in, physical and biological models will become necessary.

Research Challenges

Methods established for developing CPS must extend and scale to include the integration and interoperation of pervasive physical and biological systems. The areas of technical challenges for research and some drivers include the following:

Consumer demands and needs: An already high and still-growing cost is associated with traditional (hospital, clinic) care settings, particularly for interventions that do not demand the resources of a full-service hospital. This has led to increasing interest in alternatives such as home care, assisted living, and commoditized convenient care settings. Such emerging health care venues have the potential to become major consumers of innovative, commoditized, and cost-effective medical and laboratory technologies. A second, perhaps unexpected, driver of innovation is sports, with the growing popularity of sophisticated technologies to measure training effectiveness and athletic performance.

Networking: Future computing and networking technologies deployed in medical devices and systems are likely to be interconnected in increasingly complex open systems[10], with many heterogeneous components. Variation in the configuration of devices will be highly dynamic, determined by both economic and patient-specific medical considerations. This future will depend upon a science and technology foundation that can provide flexible and assured configuration of highly capable real-time, embedded systems with networking, data management, and control technologies. These will be expected to provide situation-appropriate levels of component autonomy, timeliness, cooperative coordination, and supervisory control, as well as high-confidence operation. At the same time, the IT substrate must integrate and manage diverse device requirements, optimize treatment delivery, and remain highly responsive to the rapidly changing requirements of the users – physician, team, and clinical care setting.

Real-Time Physiological Sensing, Control, and Feedback:

> *Sensor fusion:* Academic, government, and industry research today is exploring sensors that can be implanted or worn (e.g., attached to clothing), communicating either wirelessly or through networks woven into fabrics, and used for gait analysis, detection of falling, and monitoring for (ab)normal mobility and activity levels. A rapidly growing field of research focuses on environments that can exploit ubiquitous monitoring technologies to make assisted living and home care safer and more capable.

For example, treatment of diabetes has progressed from onerous physiological test-based methods to in-home device-based glucose measurement in patients with infusion pumps. Closed-loop control based on skin-sensing technology is on the horizon. Similarly, many other tests and studies that today are conducted "off-line" using a single or small number of samples sent to a laboratory could give way to online dynamic models obtained from continuous monitoring, which also could yield opportunities for closed-loop control.

Prosthetics: The growing demand for devices for people with debilitating injuries or disabilities is driving innovation in prosthetics of all kinds. Prosthetic devices increasingly will depend upon sophisticated information and control technology. Biomedical augmentation can be expected to expand with the advent of new biomechanical technologies and new treatment targets, such as in neural and deep brain stimulation, and retinal and cochlear implants. In long-familiar devices such as artificial limbs, hands, or feet, the potential scope for intelligent prosthetics is just beginning to be explored – e.g., the possibility that a patient can control the prosthesis through his or her own patterns of brain activity. Engineered materials and organs such as "smart skin" and an artificial pancreas are becoming realities. If such technologies are to become practical, the variety of challenges for safely and effectively controlling the interaction of the artificial and the biological must be addressed.

Minimally invasive diagnostic and intervention technologies: The current trend towards less invasive methods for obtaining biometric data and performing surgical interventions can be expected to continue. The risk of infection and collateral injury, as well as patient recovery time and care requirements all can be lowered when large surgical wounds can be avoided. Precision microsurgery is already benefiting from the march of technology, with medical device miniaturization now reaching the scale of micro- and nano- electromechanical systems (MEMS and NEMS). Devices can be snaked through blood vessels to reach areas of the heart that control contraction rhythm. The device can then, for example, perform microsurgery to induce a scar that reduces conductivity and alters the electrical signal to mitigate tachycardia, a common type of arrhythmia. Among the challenges for such devices is to avoid causing damage to the surrounding tissue and to offer precision control in the presence of varying natural motion and events in the complex human biological environment.

Control and Feedback: Increasingly sophisticated prostheses and therapeutic technologies exemplify systems that must interact well with their users or subjects. If a device has multiple functions, the system must be designed to make sure the user stays aware of, and can appropriately control, the current mode of operation. Otherwise, mode confusion may cause the user to take an erroneous action and potentially induce harm. The interaction of multiple devices operating simultaneously also must not cause hazardous conditions, and must not result in interference that prevents one or another device from properly carrying out an essential function. The patient and operator are in highly dynamic situations, in which dangerous conditions can develop rapidly. Thus the system must provide "natural," easy-to-understand modes for dealing with rapid changes and must clearly represent to the user the state of the system and the condition of the patient. For many situations, visual feedback will not be possible, and haptic feedback will provide more information.

The large number of biomarkers that may be available to improve understanding of the patient's condition will be very beneficial from a health perspective, but also may require significant technology support. For example, there may be need for data fusion and synchronization, for example, to achieve correlation of EKG, muscular, and EEG signals in real time. Critical areas for research include:

- Mode confusion causing the user to do the right thing at the wrong time o Haptic feedback
- Actuation (how you actually do what you want to do with the prosthesis) o Intelligent prosthetics
- Data fusion and synchronization (e.g., EKG-EEG correlation where signals might require real-time synchronization)
- Human in the loop
- Adaptive control

Biological and physiological systems: Simultaneous, correlated information about multiple biomarkers can be expected to yield more complete and contemporaneous assessment of a patient's condition than is generally available today. Research, invention and innovative development are required, however, to give rise to technologies that can fully exploit these new discoveries about disease processes, their physiological manifestations, and the biomarkers that are their best indicators. From a scientific and technological "push" perspective, progress in biomedical technology inevitably will be propelled by discoveries in biology and medicine; new biosensing and bioactuation inventions; advances in bio and nano materials and structures; the miniaturization, enhanced control, and increasing mobility of technologies such as mass spectrometry, ultrasound, and resonance-based imaging. Many of these are made possible by concurrent advances in the cyber technologies that enable the exploitation and precise control of physical technologies. Biological and medical advances can be expected to open new possibilities for interventions at all levels: system, organ, cellular, molecular, or even atomic.

Achieving Certifiably Dependable Medical Device Cyber-Physical Systems

Verification, Validation, and Certification

Engineers have always been challenged to provide sufficient evidence, through various methods of verification and validation (V&V), that a device or system will perform as intended. History is replete with examples of designs in all industry sectors that failed despite vast expenditures on V&V. It is tempting to say that results today are not much better than those of 20 years ago. However, that would be an arguably unfair statement in light of the orders-of-magnitude growth in complexity reflected in today's engineered systems as compared with those of the past. The fact is that manufacturers are benefiting from many research advances. This progress is reflected in their ability to design ever more complex systems with some measure of dependability.

Many of the V&V efforts to date are driven by system-life-cycle-development activities that rely primarily on methods of inspection and testing. The problem is that many of the inspection activities are "checklist"-based and subject to human factors. Similarly, testing is largely an experimental process, strongly influenced by the availability of development resources and time. Such evidence provides some confidence that a device will perform as intended.

These methods have worked reasonably well for highly constrained discrete devices that can rely on the notion of competent human intervention as an ultimate means of risk control.

Evolving the types of medical systems described in this report presents V&V challenges of unprecedented magnitude. The combination of proprietary components and third-party components of unknown pedigree creates a design space representing combinatorial assumptions (environment, timing, computing, control, communication and physical conditions) and design decisions beyond the human ability to fathom. There is an urgent need for end-to-end, principled, engineering-based (automated) design, along with V&V tools that will allow the information produced by one tool to supplement and increase the effectiveness of other tools elsewhere in the development life cycle. The aggregate artifacts of such tools serve to support the establishment of "sufficient" objectively trustworthy evidence that a medical device system will perform as intended[11].

V&V in the Presence of Change

It is rare that the design requirements for a medical system, let alone any other type of cyberphysical system, can be completely specified at the outset of a development effort. Changes in requirements and design specifications are a fact of life. The challenge is to be able to provide sufficient high-quality evidence that any system design or component change is appropriately accounted for in all system components, such as assumptions, information, timing, risks, etc.

To help minimize end-to-end testing, V& V techniques and tools are needed that can establish sufficient evidence that various system components and properties are not affected by a design or component change. A key V& V research challenge then, is to understand what is meant by the term "sufficient evidence," its properties, and how this meaning can be accepted throughout the global economy.

Certification

The workshop participants' report presents several areas of research that can enable the development of dependable medical systems. Further exploration is needed now to identify the kinds of properties and evidence derived from the proposed methods and tools that can serve as a basis for certification.

More generally, there is a need for assuring that the *interface* between design abstractions (e.g., specifications and models) and their concrete counterparts can be assessed for correctness and completeness properties. This need is absolutely critical to making assurance cases that serve to support particular medical system claims.

Safety assurance cases may be characterized as tree structures of claims, arguments, and evidence that support a "top-level" claim. These trees can become very complex. The challenge here, key to the notion of certification, is to abstract this complexity in a manner that can be *trusted* to the same level as the design abstractions and concrete counterparts they represent. The complexity represented in cyber-physical systems presents a particular challenge to assurance case abstraction. Research opportunities to facilitate trustable assurance cases are needed. For example, standard safety case patterns for various design constructs might be established.

As medical systems become ever more complex, networked, and interoperable, manufacturers will need access to open, formally composable V& V technology that relies on computational models unifying cyber and physical systems to help establish sufficient evidence.

Science and Technology R&D Needs for Designing Certifiably Dependable Medical Device Cyber-Physical Systems

Scientific Foundations for Cyber-Physical Systems

Today, foundations are lacking that could enable both the design and assurance of medical device cyber-physical systems. Many different facets of these systems will have to be analyzed including the environmental, structural, kinematic, biologic, chemical, and thermal interactions as well as the logical interactions of the controlled device(s) with users, operators, and patient status.

The analytic tools needed for design and certification will need to span the relevant theories in mathematics, dynamics, and control; sensor data fusion and information management; communication; real-time computing; and hardware and systems software platform technology. Unification and interoperation of theories and tools will be needed to support high-confidence development and certification.

Open systems demand interoperability of the constituent components. To date, we do not have open systems foundations for a broad range of medical technologies, a lack that may inhibit the scope of innovation in medicine and biomedical technology.

Foundations of both development and assurance are needed for open networked control of cyber-physical systems.

Foundations for evidence-based design and certification are needed that replace indirect (process- and best practice-based) certification with methods for direct (product-oriented) evaluation and assurance. The growing suite of verification technologies needs to be open and interoperable to enable methods that are appropriate for each assurance task and components that can be easily configured or interchanged.

R&D Needs in Design and Implementation Capability and Infrastructure for Cyber-Physical Systems

The workshop participants' report recommends research to create new robust, embedded, real-time, networked system infrastructure for medical device software and systems. The workshop identified significant gaps in design and implementation capability to meet the objectives of reliable, privacy-preserving, cost-effective, personalized, and high-quality health care. The gaps were examined further in the subsequent HCMDSS/PnP workshop.

The objectives for improving health care are extremely challenging technically. Current efforts to address interoperability, for example, are at the level of network connectivity. This will not be sufficient. New systems support capability also will be needed to orchestrate the interactions between devices and between devices and human users, and to assure that the device actions can be coordinated and carried out in real time. This is not merely a software problem, but fundamentally involves the control design of devices and systems. Current methods for analyzing issues such as the timing characteristics of software, control performance, hazard analysis, and failure modes and effects cannot simply be applied to the individual components. Composite systems, particularly ones that interact with the nondeterministic actions of humans, may exhibit unexpected emergent behaviors. New assurance methods will be required to evaluate the new system integration or coordination capabilities and to support the safety and security implications for the interacting devices and the system as a whole.

As noted in the workshop report, today's closed and vertically integrated systems present technical and economic obstacles to rapid uptake of biomedical discoveries and inventions.

The HCSS agencies recommend that a strategic R&D focus on high-confidence networking and IT for the design, implementation, and certification of ***open medical technologies*** *be undertaken, both to meet the goals of cost-effective, tailored, and patient-specific treatment, and to spur a level of device and systems innovation that can sustain a competitive global role for the U.S. in biomedical technology.*

Modeling, Design, and Implementation Technology

The 2006 workshop report identified research needs in three major areas, including:

Patient modeling and simulation
Medical device software development

Model-based design frameworks

The 2007 workshop extended this discussion to consider highly configurable diagnostic and treatment settings.

Participants in both workshops recommended increased R&D in patient-based modeling that can explain the interactions of organs and systems of the human body. This research would go beyond traditional computational data-analysis methods; it would attempt to build and validate constituent organ and system models that could be used in a compositional modeling environment to represent contemporaneous functioning of systems and the patient as a whole. In embedded software development, the workshops recommend R&D in technology to enable formal and model-based analysis, design, and implementation of open medical-device and system software. These recommendations focus on the need for component-based design and system integration. In the area of design automation, the workshop series presents arguments for developing a model-based tool chain for semantic integration of these systems.

A strategic focus on R&D in compositional modeling and design is needed to address the open systems needs and to bridge the jointly cyber and physical aspects of this complex systems problem. The aggregate of patient physiology (including functions and pathologies of diverse organs and systems), the medical devices for diagnosis and therapeutic interventions affecting these systems, and the architecture and overall control of the sensing and treatment system constitute a complex system. R&D is needed to resolve fundamental issues underlying the composition and integration of cyber-physical device and infrastructure technologies through semantics-based and model-based tool chains that represent and resolve both logical and physical interoperability. *We also concur with the workshop recommendation that a key area of research needed to enable this vision is the incremental certified composition of certified components. This is expected to contribute to both early discovery of problems (hence safer designs and implementations) and higher confidence to support the acceptance of systems by users and regulators.*

Infrastructure for Medical-Device Integration and Interoperation

The workshop series emphasizes the need for infrastructure that supports active fault detection, isolation, and recovery for fail-safe support of systems of devices. *We recommend increased emphasis on R&D that will contribute to more capable technology platforms that monitor their own (possibly distributed) operational status and protect applications from infrastructure-induced failures.*

Networking

The workshops posited scenarios in which devices cooperate over (possibly wireless) networks to provide treatment and care in new settings. The "operating room of the future" concept, for example, envisions an all-wireless, configurable operating room. Home care would be enhanced by technology to monitor and treat chronic conditions of elderly, convalescing, or disabled patients, and to report any transition to acute care requirements. The workshops outlined needs for "critical infrastructure" that can enable such concepts. Networking that can accommodate configurations of many (often life- or safety-critical) devices is one component of such infrastructure.

Increased emphasis is needed across the networking research landscape on the requirements of distributed devices that must communicate, control, and interact under strict timing, determinism, energy, and (re)configurability constraints. Some progress has been made, but great variation exists across sectors. Commercial standards such as CAN and FlexRay prescribe functionality for real-time networks used in automotive, aviation, and process- control systems. The ARINC 664 standard prescribes a deterministic Ethernet-based databus for aviation. A standard for timed Ethernet, IEEE 1588, is emerging. *Although these standards are broadly relevant, we agree that the need and opportunity exist to address the particular safety, privacy, and security challenges of device networks for preventive, chronic, and acute health care.*

R&D is needed that can contribute to open, non-proprietary interoperability standards and provide advanced capabilities for managing the safety, security, and privacy aspects of communication. This includes the latency and real-time, fault-tolerance, and device registration and configurability requirements imposed in an open medical device network infrastructure that includes wide-area networking. Among the many considerations for medical networks are the potential for electromagnetic frequency (EMF, e.g. radio frequency) interference among wireless devices and between wireless transmitters (e.g., radios, routers) and medical device emissions; network and transmitter contention for energy resources and interactive power management; preservation of network connectivity and quality of service in an active EMF and complex physical environment; time-awareness; and other special requirements such as mobility and active localization.

Real-time Operating Systems and Middleware

One-size-fits-all operating systems will not suffice for all medical applications, although some industry-specific solutions do exist to address particular issues. For example, ARINC 653 is an aviation standard for real-time operating systems that provides spatial and temporal separation to assure that applications do not conflict in their use of system resources. The workshops identify important gaps. For example, middleware that is based upon best-effort scheduling may meet requirements for electronic health records but not for device-to-device interaction. Plug-and-play may place new demands, such as:

- New principles for virtualization in a complex, heterogeneous physical world
- New services such as schedulers that can accommodate both synchronous and reactive system needs
- Dynamic scheduling with both hard and soft real-time guarantees
- Reconfigurable fault tolerance and redundancy management
- Dynamic support for resource isolation
- Execution control concepts for cooperating, multimodal embedded systems
- Drivers for increasingly complex sensing and actuation devices and platform technologies; device attestation, calibration, and device health monitoring
- Security services that are compatible with real-time and embedded systems requirements
- Network stacks with support for mobility

Support for new hardware substrates, including reconfigurable hardware and reconfigurable networks
Distributed coordination services

Real-Time Hardware/Software Platforms

Trends towards dependence on configurable architectures such as field-programmable gate arrays (FPGAs) and perhaps eventually multicore system-on-chip (SoC) architectures, where each core is an FPGA, must also be addressed. It will be necessary to certify that implementations provide the specified functionality and satisfy non-functional constraints on properties such as timing, energy consumption, and thermal gain. Resource virtualization can be expected to be an increasing challenge because of the interactive and interdependent operation of the constituent platform configurations. In the much longer term, new computational and networking platforms may be influenced by outcomes from nanotechnology and biomolecular computing research, possibly exhibiting even greater variability that must be masked or controlled.

At the same time, these architectures present new opportunities to support capabilities such as extended built-in self-testing on the hardware platform, system-level device health monitoring, fault isolation and recovery, hardware-level security implementation, and device attestation. New concepts such as timed-instruction-set architectures and delay-insensitive system architectures currently are being explored, in a quest for hardware support that can provide determinism for complex, interactive systems of devices. *Research is needed on additional concepts that seek to advance capability and dependability at the platform level.*

Sensing, Control, and Coordination Concepts

The workshop report identifies closed-loop control of devices as an emerging trend and notes that coordination among multiple devices must be provided. This is a challenge that must be addressed at all levels of a system or configuration of cooperating medical devices. There is some prior research upon which to build. Open control platforms have been explored at a rudimentary level. Distributed control has received substantial attention over the past several years. Hybrid control theory has sought to unify the discrete (logical, switched, or event- driven) aspects of control with the continuous behavior and recurrent control relation of the physical system. Model-predictive control (both conventional and hybrid) has improved the performance and safety of individual systems. Limited mechanisms such as software interlocks have been devised to limit or force concurrent operation of cooperating devices.

However, the challenges of coordinated control in either a vertically integrated or an open plug-and-play setting, where the effects of multiple-device operation are coupled in a human subject, far exceed the reach of today's science and technology. Compositional abstractions for sensing and control are needed to underpin next-generation supervisory control. A central challenge is to arrange for cooperative control across hierarchies of devices and subsystems, and to do so in the face of diverse and possibly changing configurations. Change may also arise suddenly due to a change in patient status, requiring coordinated response from multiple devices. Some devices may be autonomous and others operated by humans, requiring a mixed-initiative strategy for managing control authority in the system.

In such complex and changing environments, learning technology may hold promise as a means to help in acquiring models of prevailing or changing system dynamics – an important step beyond state estimation. However, suitability, dependability, and certifiability must be established for all technologies intended for use in this complex environment, operating under the real-time and other constraints posed by the dynamic physical and computational context, and including appropriate representation of uncertainty.

Assurance Capability

Supporting Technology

The workshop report emphasizes the need for "design for certifiably dependable systems" to supersede today's process-based, post hoc certification methods. We agree with this finding and that of the National Academies study, *Software for Dependable Systems: Sufficient Evidence*? The needed technology focus should be support for evaluation capabilities that pervade the design process, not simply support for post hoc evaluation of the system. The production of evidence that the system is properly constructed, functions as intended, and operates safely and securely, is a second key focus. High confidence must be sought through a combination of lightweight (easily useable and sometimes approximate) methods, as well as heavier-weight methods that can deliver rigor and completeness where that is required. *Research is needed to provide a new generation of analysis, synthesis, and composition and integration technology for cyber-physical systems such as medical devices and systems.*

Analysis Concepts and Tools

The view has faded that all verification must be conducted by an automatic or semi-automatic theorem prover, proving "correctness" of the whole system and taking hours or days. Verification technology is making new strides in areas such as lightweight methods for the analysis of software or system before it is executed ("static analysis") and checking the system for flaws that may violate the software or system specification ("model checking"). Advances have been made in abstraction, such as the construction of simplified behavioral models from software, or the extraction of predicates about properties of a system from lower- level models. Model checking is a generalized technique that is capable of scouring very large state spaces for undesirable conditions and assuring that the system or software cannot reach such conditions. Static analysis and checking techniques for software are achieving rapid advances in capability, and are now widely used for bug-finding and more comprehensive analysis of industrial software.

We agree with the workshop report that further substantial research is needed to achieve comprehensive end-to-end analysis and checking capability for the wide range of (possibly interacting) properties critical to system performance, behavior, function, safety, and security.

Synthesis Concepts and Tools

Much of today's medical software is generated as a by-product of mathematical modeling tools. These tools typically make a rather direct translation of the mathematical formulas in the system simulation into code (usually C code). Code quality is a pervasive concern. Although some modeling systems provide real-time analysis for various hardware platforms, the capabilities are limited and focus on single system requirements. For complex cyber-physical systems, a great deal of software (both application and system software) is required that has nothing to do with the mathematical algorithm. Synthesis of the behavioral and interactive aspects of a system (of systems) currently lags far behind in the level of both scientific understanding and technical support.

Composition/Integration Tools

To achieve useful technologies based on solid scientific foundations, the current fragmented methods must be replaced by much more expressive and interoperable concepts for component, property, and system representation. Model-based design takes a step in this direction, seeking to produce designs that have rich semantics based on both physical and computational systems concepts. Synthesis tools and the technology base must have a coherent shared semantic interface. However, the class of models (computational, physical, properties) available today is impoverished relative to the systems we are seeking to build.

As highlighted in the workshop report, research is needed towards open systems interface checking. This should include tools (e.g., based on static analysis and model checking) that can check the interoperability of components and generate composable evidence for their properties relevant to medical technologies (mutually exclusive or simultaneous operation, non-interference, timeliness). Many of these properties may be broadly applicable to CPS, not only to the medical device domain. Research concepts such as "assume/guarantee" reasoning, which describes the desired behavior of composite systems based upon the constituent subsystems, should continue to be extended to provide "composable evidence" that would integrate both the functional components and the evidence about their individual correct functioning and properties, producing both the designed product and evidence that the composite system is correct.

An Open Verification Technology Perspective

Interoperability of formal reasoning methods has been advanced through a focus on smaller (e.g., property-based) theories that can be combined under a single logical framework. Counterexamples, which can be harvested from failed attempts to prove properties correct, have been found very useful in illuminating problem areas, not only after the system is complete but also during its development. However, much remains to be done. The techniques described above on analysis, synthesis, and integration are individual methods and are not organized for easy, coherent use; nor are their interfaces couched in terms of systems problems. The research community argues (and we agree) that tools both for functional synthesis and analysis of the system and for synthesis of evidence must be integrated semantically. The idea of an "evidential tool bus" has been described that provides for transmission of the synthesis, analysis, and checking artifacts among tools, to be composed at the same time the components themselves are assembled.

Evidence-Based Certification Technology

The research community has proposed a new approach to "scientific certification" or "direct assurance," in which the critical properties of the product system are formally scrutinized to the extent possible. Certification is based on evidence produced in this process, ideally evidence that is extracted rigorously using analysis tools, or provided as an adjunct to synthesis or integration in an open verification environment. Active discussion is occurring on the potential use of assurance cases, which are organized collections of claims, arguments, and evidence that establish the safety or security of a system. The FDA held a workshop in February 2008 that brought assurance case experts from FDA and academia together with representatives of industry organizations. The assurance case concept was well received; future meetings are planned to explore its challenges for industry and regulators.

Human-Machine Interaction

Medical devices and systems interact with humans in two ways: humans as operators ("users") and humans as subjects. Sometimes, the human is both user and subject. We agree with the general view that device and systems technology based on broad classes of subjects are often less effective than those that can be tailored to the individual user. Patient-specific modeling and simulation is needed to enable adaptive and patient-specific therapies. New approaches to designing interfaces are also needed that enable natural interaction and sustain: a) shared human and cyber understanding of the current and possible or predictable states (both normal and failure) of the system, b) agreement on actions that can be taken, and c) sharing of authority between humans and medical devices.

A Holistic Cyber-Physical Systems Perspective

As medical technology moves to smaller scales, where cellular and even molecular dynamics prevail, new opportunities for deeply integrated sensing and control are emerging. At the same time, growing understanding of systems biology may give rise to new strategies for medical technology that exploit computation-driven sensing and control interactions with "systems of systems," the interacting complex of mechanisms spanning the cellular level up to the organs and macro systems of the human body.

To enable the holistic understanding that researchers and industry will need to build the next generations of medical device cyber-physical systems, barriers must fall that currently divide the underpinning disciplines: medicine, discrete and continuous mathematics of dynamics and control; real-time computation and communication; medical robotics; learning; computational models and the supporting systems design and implementation technologies; and formal and algorithmic methods for checking and reasoning about system properties.

Increasingly, multidisciplinary science, engineering, and education practices will be required to deal with the inherent complexity of the advanced medical systems described here and their life-critical technical challenges.

Collaboration Challenges and Strategies to Address Medical Device R&D Needs

Federal R&D Interests in Medical Device Technology

The Federal government has a direct interest in promoting comprehensive examination of the development, deployment, and use of medical technologies. One mission of the FDA's Center for Devices and Radiological Health is evaluating the safety and effectiveness of medical devices for market, including those that are IT-controlled. The missions of NSF and NIH include supporting short-, medium-, and long-term research and development of bioengineering and medical technology. NSF also supports long-term research in cyber-physical systems, spanning real-time embedded systems, control systems, networking, robotics, devices and materials, software, and assurance methods. NIST's non-regulatory mission – developing and promoting measurement, standards, and technology in concert with industries and research laboratories – affects both research and implementation across all device domains. NIST's Manufacturing and Engineering Laboratory develops and supports performance metrics and standards for manufacturing technology, robotics, and industrial control systems; its Information Technology Laboratory also supports projects relevant to medical software and systems including security, certification, user interfaces, software diagnostics, conformance testing, and network research.

Other Federal agencies, such as the Department of Health and Human Services and its Centers for Disease Control, have broad charges associated with watching over the health and welfare of the nation's citizens. The current Federal initiative for a Nationwide Health Information Network (NHIN) has the goals of informing clinical practice, particularly in remote areas; interconnecting clinicians to foster collaboration; personalizing health care; and streamlining the monitoring of public health to improve the health of the overall population. The initiative envisions a complete electronic health record (EHR) for every patient at any point of service. The EHR would provide practitioners with the patient's medical history, remind the patient of treatment steps, and track outcomes and quality of health care delivery.

Realizing these systems will require R&D gains on multiple fronts. The Veterans' Administration (VA), for example, has encountered challenges in correctly correlating clinical data and images with patient records, a significant issue because of the immense number of archived images involved. The VA has a particular interest in the unique identification of data and in validating the conformance of medical devices during use, as well as in surgical data and support systems to eliminate "wrong patient," "wrong surgery," "wrong site" situations.

The Department of Defense's Telemedicine and Technology Research Center (TATRC) is involved in all aspects of system integration, demonstration and evaluation of new communications and information systems technologies to improve health care for soldiers and all DoD beneficiaries. Today, TATRC is charged with managing both a general research/development program and specific advanced technology projects in multiple areas including: knowledge engineering; combat trauma training systems; distance learning; computer- aided instruction; medical imaging; medical data fusion and distribution; image-guided therapies; minimally invasive therapies; advanced diagnostic and therapeutic systems; wireless medical systems; teleconsultation systems; robotics; medical modeling and simulation; and physiological sensors.

Other agencies that do not have mission responsibilities for medical applications nonetheless have a keen interest in high-confidence technologies. NSA, for example, has a focus on identifying and addressing crucial issues for the design, certification, and operation of extremely secure and reliable software and systems. NSA's concerns include many of those involved in medical device cyber-physical systems, including the increasing complexity of critical systems, the accelerating product-development cycles due to market pressures, and the effort, time, and cost of certification processes for critical systems.

Federal R&D Investments for Medical Device Technology

Federal research in cyber-physical and embedded systems has been pursued in a variety of programs over the past decade, initially in DARPA's Quorum, Software Enabled Control (SEC), Model-Based Integration of Embedded Software (MoBIES), Program Composition for Embedded Systems (PCES), and Adaptive and Reflective Middleware Systems (ARMS) programs. Some continuing progress has been achieved under the NSF Information Technology Research (ITR), Emerging Frontiers in Research and Innovation (EFRI), and Embedded and Hybrid Systems (EHS) programs, and more recently, Cyber-Physical Systems (CPS) program; NIST's Advanced Technology Program (now Technology Innovation Program); and DoD Multidisciplinary University Research Initiative (MURI) programs. Advances through these programs and across the networking and IT landscape place the nation in good position to tackle, through a focused R&D effort, the fundamental challenges in developing high-confidence medical cyber-physical systems that can transform 21st century health care.

We agree with the President's Council of Advisors on Science and Technology that robust R&D in cyber-physical systems is critical for maintaining U.S. technological and economic leadership in the years ahead.[12] *The HCSS agencies have an unprecedented opportunity to collaboratively embark upon a larger-scale strategic effort in this area.*

Coordination Challenges

The following considerations should be addressed in shaping a multiagency Federal research agenda for this effort:

> Agencies differ in their R&D horizons (long-term/short-term/transition and standards), research management strategy (project-oriented programs, large-scale grants-based programs, centers), investment strategies (primarily intramural vs. extramural), funding instruments (contracts, grants), constituency (industry, academia, mixed), and funding allocation timelines (six-month, one-year, multi-

year). Matching R&D horizons to agency roles is critical to a successful interagency effort.

No one agency covers the full spectrum of needed research. Often, the mechanisms for funding a science or technology area reside in many cross-cutting programs or in small programs with highly specific funding constraints and objectives (research programs, advanced technology programs, Small Business Innovation Research grants (SBIRs), NSF's Integrative Graduate Education and Research Traineeship [IGERT], education). Cooperation and coordination among agencies can be used to leverage individual efforts in pursuing larger R&D goals.

A broad mix of research funding strategies appears needed to stimulate innovation and transition. This could be enabled by cooperative efforts and funding strategies that span multiple agencies and programs.

University Research

The current university research portfolio in the areas of real-time and embedded systems, robotics, sensor nets, control theory, adaptive systems, learning and game theories, operating systems and middleware, and formal methods; verification and analysis of embedded systems and software; networking; and engineering of materials, sensors, and other devices is of high quality but limited scale. Further, innovation-driven research occurring at universities is not being adequately tapped by industry. Universities are leading in the development of evidence-based artifacts and measures that would benefit both industry and regulators. The research community, as noted in the HCMDSS workshop report and others, calls for expanded engagement that spans academia, government, and industry.

Industry R&D in Medical Device Technology

Industrial research necessarily is driven by time-to-market concerns; much of its focus is on the development of new medical technologies or improvements in the capabilities of existing devices and systems. Profit margins and economic pressures, such as time-driven return on investments and competition with leading high-technology producers in other countries, such as Germany, Japan, and the Netherlands[13], tend to focus industry investments on the development of devices that create new market opportunities. Within these constraints, industry efforts continue to produce innovations such as deep-brain stimulation devices. These require large investments for research and prototyping, product development, and safety evaluation. Recognizing both the unique capabilities and the competitive landscape within which industrial entities operate is critical to establishing productive public-private partnerships.

Federal-Private Sector Collaboration Issues and Strategies

Incentives are needed to promote effective cooperation between government, industry, and academia to build the underpinning networking and information technology frameworks for the open, interoperable systems future described here.

New approaches to intellectual property (IP) will be necessary, for example, to enable robust interaction among industry, academia, and government. The establishment of an open experimental platform for use by researchers to investigate technologies for integrating medical device systems could circumvent some of the IP issues. Such a platform would contain design artifacts, including reference models and scenarios about the use of various medical devices, so that researchers could obtain empirical feedback on their ideas about real systems.

It will also be necessary to develop nonthreatening means of accurate error reporting in medical devices and systems. Engineering high-confidence technology requires feedback on its actual use in the intended setting, and errors, anomalies, malfunctions, and the like are essential data points. We are able to report and track device incidents (accidents, malfunctions, apparent problems, and other categories of adverse events) but reporting, tracking, publicizing, and interpreting the root causes of device incidents across manufacturers is problematic due to litigation risks. The use of aggregate or case-blind data could provide at least limited solutions to these problems. Approaches such as the black box flight recorder used in aircraft and automated system health maintenance strategies ("zero-failure systems") being explored for automotive and aviation systems also are needed to capture, integrate, and correlate data on medical device and system failures, malfunctions, and degraded operation. These are multidisciplinary and multifaceted problems that would benefit from collaborative engagement by researchers, industry, and government regulators.

Testbeds and Other Mechanisms

Federal agency workshop participants agree with the workshop report that there is a critical need for open-system experimental platforms and standardized research data sets (that include protection for intellectual property) to foster collaboration between academic, industry, and Federal researchers. Also needed are specific mechanisms to foster collaboration. *A study on how best to establish such testbeds, including a plan for implementation, could light the way forward in pursuing this recommendation.*

Other Opportunities for Collaboration

The following are examples, by category, of challenge problems that would benefit from united efforts to develop exemplary solutions.

Models

> Process models from clinicians and their workflows, analyses of change effects, and measures of system quality and performance that can support a systems engineering approach

Nominal models that specify safe and effective functionality and appropriate use for a class of devices

Tools

Tools supporting compositional analysis, together with component-based designs based upon formal models of medical devices, control algorithms, and workflows of medical practice, and producing design-based evidence that is useful for certification

Formal, integrated, end-to-end, model-based development frameworks including requirements gathering, specification, design, simulation, and verification and dealing with composition, evolution, and change throughout the product lifecycle

Sensing, Monitoring, and Control

A networked sensing and control system on a mobile distributed population with more than 1,000 nodes

Configurable communication, sensing, and control systems for specific scenarios such as emergency-room (ER) or geriatric care

Integrated, portable, preoperative and postoperative monitoring systems for evaluating the medical status of a patient in both traditional and non-traditional points of care

An integrated health care system of systems architecture for distributed monitoring and control for uses such as hospitals, civilian emergency response, 911, or combat settings, where detailed medical status of patients or victims requiring or under care may be provided to monitoring, dispatch, or command centers

Systems

An initial set of publicly available model application problems and a corresponding suite of coherent protocols designed and rigorously specified and verified for correctness and compatibility

Medical-device software and systems that can prevent misuse by caregivers, adapt to changing patient conditions, and be safely used in closed-loop situations

Quality of Service (QoS)-aware, fault-tolerant, certified middleware infrastructure suitable for pervasive use in medical systems of systems, guaranteeing QoS, safety constraints, security and privacy, and assured by validation and certification

VV&C

Develop medical-practice-driven design and validation, including metrics for usability evaluation and user-centered design methods

Develop certified components as commodities

Gain a fundamental understanding of how to design protocols that make certification easier and how to develop an evidence-based, technology-aware certification process

Reorient the certification process toward component-based certification

Devise the medical-device equivalent of a "black box" flight recorder with audit capability to trace the circumstances leading up to untoward events

Testbed Standards

A suite of model interoperability standards
An assessment of technical deficiencies observed in today's medical IT devices and systems and identification of design opportunities that would yield improved care

APPENDICES

Appendix 1. Agencies Contributing to This Report

Agency for Healthcare Research and Quality (AHRQ)
Food and Drug Administration (FDA)
National Coordination Office for the NITRD Program
National Institute of Standards and Technology (NIST)
National Security Agency (NSA)
National Science Foundation (NSF)
National Transportation Safety Board (NT SB)

Appendix 2. Participation in HCSS Coordination Activities

HCSS Coordinating Group Co-Chairs
Helen Gill, NSF
Brad Martin, NSA
Albert Wavering, NIST

HCSS Member and Participating Agencies as of April 2008
Air Force Research Laboratory (AFRL)
Air Force Office of Scientific Research (AFOSR)
Army Research Office (ARO)
Department of Energy (DOE)
Federal Aviation Administration (FAA)
Food and Drug Administration (FDA)
National Aeronautics and Space Administration (NASA)
National Institute of Standards and Technology (NIST)
National Institutes of Health (NIH) National Science Foundation (NSF)
National Security Agency (NSA)
Office of the Secretary of Defense (OSD)

NCO/NITRD
Frankie Denise King, HCSS Technical Coordinator

Appendix 3. HCMDSS Workshop Participants' Report

Report on the High-Confidence Medical-Device Software and Systems (HCMDSS) Workshop

February 6, 2006

Report Authors

Insup Lee, University of Pennsylvania, Co-Chair
George Pappas, University of Pennsylvania, Co-Chair
Rance Cleaveland, University of Maryland
John Hatcliff, Kansas State University
Bruce Krogh, Carnegie Mellon University
Peter Lee, Carnegie Mellon University
Harvey Rubin, University of Pennsylvania
Lui Sha, University of Illinois at Urbana Champaign

Executive Summary

Background and Scope

The United States spends about 16% of its gross domestic product on health care—twice the average of most European nations (Health Information Leadership Panel, Final Report, Department of Health and Human Services, March 2005). The rapidly increasing use of software to control medical devices makes the development and production of medical-device software and systems a crucial issue, both for the U.S. economy and for ensuring safe advances in health care delivery. Several federal agencies are interested in identifying the research necessary to improve the design, certification, and operation of medical-device software and systems. The ultimate goal is better and more cost effective medical care.

On June 2 and 3, 2005, the High-Confidence Medical Device Software and Systems (HCMDSS) workshop was held in Philadelphia. An HCMDSS Workshop Planning Meeting (WPM) had been held on November 16 and 17, 2004, in Arlington, Virginia. The WPM was sponsored by the NITRD federal agencies that participate in the HCSS Coordination Group (CG), including FDA, NIST, NSA, and NSF, along with the National Coordination Office for NITRD. Sixty experts participated in the planning meeting, including those in government and industry information technology, software engineers, medical doctors, nurses, and academic researchers.

The objective of the workshop was to build on the work accomplished at the planning meeting and to identify additional challenges and approaches from other constituencies. More than 90 experts from academia, medical sectors, industry, and government attended the workshop. They represented a complete mix of the relevant stakeholders—including researchers, developers, certifiers, and users—who can help identify emerging systems and assurance needs. This report, a tangible outcome of the workshop, prioritizes recommendations by using a roadmap to determine what, when, and how priorities should be addressed over identified time frames.

Purposes and Format of Workshop

The purpose of the HCMDSS workshop was to provide a working forum for leaders and visionaries from industry, research laboratories, academia, and government concerned with medical devices. The main goal was to develop a roadmap for overcoming crucial issues and challenges facing the design, manufacture, certification, and use of medical-device software and systems. An additional goal was to identify and form a sustainable research and development (R&D) community for the advancement of HCMDSS. Of particular interest was the crystallization of technology needs and promising research directions that could revolutionize the way HCMDSS are designed, produced, and validated in the future but that are beyond the range of today's devices because of time-to-market pressures and short-term R&D practices.

The HCMDSS workshop included plenary and panel discussions and breakout sessions. The panels and breakout sessions addressed the following six issues essential to HCMDSS:

1. **Distributed Sensing and Control in Networked Medical-Device Systems.** The networking of medical devices for distributed sensing and control can occur at many levels. Although ad hoc growth of network applications for medical devices has occurred, today's commercial off-the-shelf technologies (COTS) do not produce highly distributed medical-device systems with guarantees of security, privacy, robustness, interoperability, extensibility, mobility, and general patient safety. Research is needed to create medical-device networks with those features and to enable the diffusion of new sensing and control technologies as they become available.

2. **Embedded Real-Time Networked System Infrastructure for Medical-Device Software and Systems (MDSS).** The next generation of medical systems is envisioned to be a ubiquitous network of networked systems for secure, reliable, privacy-preserving, and cost- effective personalized high-quality health care. It will be a network that improves the quality of life. Although networks of networked medical devices hold many promises and possibilities, they also create challenges.

3. **Patient Modeling and Simulation.** Modeling has proved its value in many industries, such as aerospace, automotive, and chemical plants. It has fostered novel product development, better safety parameters, cost-effective development phases, and ultimately achieving regulatory approval. In the medical-practice domain, modcling and simulation will improve outcomes and quality of care and will provide better utilization of health care costs—with improvements in prevention, intervention, and maximal use of the electronic health record (EHR).

4. **Medical-Device Software Development.** Many medical devices are, essentially, embedded systems. As such, software is often a fundamental, albeit not always obvious, part of a device's functionality. This means that any safety and regulatory requirements for medical devices necessarily call for rigorous methods of software development to ensure reliability and to protect the public health. Exactly how to accomplish that is a major question, particularly because devices and systems are becoming increasingly complicated and interconnected. We have reached the point where testing as the primary way to gain confidence in a system is impractical or ineffective. Furthermore, requirements and specifications based on medical practice are needed in order to ensure that devices will perform appropriately.

5. **Foundations for Integrating Medical-Device Systems and Models.** Advances in computing are instrumental in the development of novel diagnostic and therapeutic equipment and procedures and of widely accessible medical-record systems. Although diagnostic and treatment systems have advanced significantly, they do not work well together. Systemic inefficiencies in health care delivery grossly inflate costs and contribute to avoidable medical errors that degrade patient care.

6. **Verification, Validation, and Certification.** Verification and validation (V&V) tasks required for the approval of medical devices play a significant role in enabling the FDA to carry out its mandate of approving only "safe and effective" medical devices. Unfortunately, many industry observers believe that we are approaching the limits of current device certification processes. As devices grow more and more complex and rely much more on embedded software to achieve critical functionality, existing certification processes are being stressed. The results: higher development costs for manufacturers, longer time to market, and increased chances of device failure—with associated recall or liability costs.

Each working group that participated in the workshop was asked to summarize the state of the art in practice, development, and research in its area, and to identify R&D needs and challenges, along with a roadmap to address the needs and challenges. This report, the full document of the HCMDSS workshop, includes the Executive Summary and six working-group summaries.

Findings from the workshop are summarized below.

Current State of Affairs and R&D Needs

Advances in computing, networking, sensing, and medical-device technology are enabling the dramatic proliferation of diagnostic and therapeutic devices. Those devices range from advanced imaging machines to minimally invasive surgical techniques, from camera-pills to doctor-on-achip, from infusion pumps to implantable heart devices. Although advances in standalone diagnostic and treatment systems have been accelerating steadily, the lack of proper integration and interoperation of those systems produces systemic inefficiencies in health care delivery. This inflates costs and contributes to avoidable medical errors that degrade patient care. The use of software that controls medical devices to overcome these problems is inevitable and will ensure safe advances in health care delivery. The crucial issue, however, is the cost-effective development and production of reliable and safe medical-device software and systems.

Here are several observations about the state of the art in medical-device software development.

Medical-Device Software Development. Designing bug-free software is difficult, especially in complex devices that may be used in unanticipated contexts. Existing practices have worked as well as they have because industry V&V personnel and regulators take their jobs seriously.

Large-Scale, Complex Devices Stress Current Best Practices. We are still challenged by large-scale, complex devices, such as proton therapy facilities. For these types of devices, the validation procedures and test cases can number in the hundreds of thousands. The burden of validation—in time and costs—slows the time to bring devices to market. Engineers often feel overwhelmed by complexity. Because of time-to-deliver pressure and a lack of properly trained software engineers, the development of HCMDSS has, with very few exceptions, not kept pace with software assurance techniques practiced in other safety-critical domains, such as avionics.

Integration of MDSS. Industry is doing fairly well at integrating products developed by a single manufacturer. Such integrations are largely proceeding ad hoc, however, without standardized integration mechanisms that are commonplace in other domains, such as the highly successful and widely used universal serial bus (USB) from the personal-computer domain. Because the number of medical devices and systems that are to be networked and integrated is increasing significantly, we must develop standards and regulations for medical- device integration.

Device Interference and Interoperation. Caregivers and clinical engineers report that as devices proliferate and as sophistication and connectivity in hospitals increase, we are becoming lost in a swirl of technology, and we face unanticipated interference between devices. A concerted effort to address interoperability has begun, aiming to develop plugand-play interoperability standards for the operating room of the future. So far the main concern has been network standards; other essential issues, such as quality of service (QoS) and semantic compatibility for interoperation, have not yet been addressed. Also, we need to conduct a systematic study of device interference during integration.

Approval and Certification. FDA device approval centers on a process-driven approach, in which manufacturers obtain approval by showing that they have carried out the process of applying established quality assurance techniques to certain levels of coverage, such as manual code inspections and testing. As a whole, the medical industry does reasonably well in developing and approving standalone devices that have moderate complexity and are based on mature technology. But when considering larger devices with relatively complex functionality, the time and costs associated with V&V tasks such as test generation and execution cause researchers to lose confidence in their ability to bring safe and effective devices to market.

It is important to consider the effectiveness and already high costs of development and certification processes in the context of rapid advances in technology that have fundamentally changed the way many informational, financial, and scientific services are provided. Although technological advances have contributed to a steady increase in the quality of health care, and although FDA approval processes have mostly kept pace, we now seem to be on the cusp of the types of revolutionary changes in health care systems that have transformed other sectors of the nation's infrastructure and economy. Such changes call for a paradigm shift in the development and certification of medical-device software and systems.

For example, pervasive networking will enable the integration of national networks, regional health care centers, local hospitals and clinics, the offices of primary-care physicians, home computing, and body-area networks. The health care IT infrastructure will focus on "systems of systems," based on architectures built around middleware, that integrate and blend monitoring and treatment devices. Networks will stream data into medical records that are automatically mined to extract knowledge that drives a host of activities, such as automated treatment and dosing and long-term research into human health and the effectiveness of treatment.

For health care providers, operating rooms and other venues of diagnosis and treatment will shift from a collection of fixed monolithic devices to plug-and-play components that enable flexible and rapid reconfiguration of diagnostic, recording, and treatment systems. Advances in minimally invasive medical robotics and real-time high-speed networks will make telemedicine and robotic surgery technologies widely available. As generations of technology-savvy health care consumers enter retirement, they will embrace—and even demand—sophisticated home care monitoring, treatment, and record systems integrated with national information databases (such as prescription-drug information systems) and hospital and primary-care systems.

These envisioned innovations hold great promise, but they will render current MDSS development and certification processes obsolete. End-user demands inevitably exceed the capability of existing MDSS. Unless new certification technologies are developed and unless development and certification processes undergo a paradigm shift, innovation will be stifled, because manufacturers and regulators will find the development of HCMDSS systems too costly—or we will see dramatic increases in security breaches and harmful incidents due to device malfunction.

R&D Challenges

The cross-cutting nature of medical-device design—transcending the informational, physical, and medical worlds—along with the possibility of a nationwide networked medical system that actively monitors and regulates the health of our nation's citizens, raises immense scientific and technological R&D challenges for the IT, medical, and regulatory communities. Here are some of the challenges we envision for the next ten years:

System Integration. As we embrace a "plug and play" vision of medical-device networks in future digital hospitals and digital homes, we must collectively facilitate the development of medical-device systems and coordinate them with the development of standards for the architecture and communication of interoperable plug-and-play (PnP) device networks. Achieving that while achieving quality-of-service levels that ensure system and patient safety on the one hand and patient security and privacy on the other hand is a great challenge.

Critical Infrastructure. As we head toward an environment where all patients are constantly monitored and actively plugged into a nationwide medical information network, we are creating a new critical infrastructure that will literally monitor the nation's health. We need new methods to ensure the safety and security of that network, particularly methods involving the active use of information for medical purposes. In the presence of abnormal conditions, or attacks, the performance of the system must degrade gracefully and safely, and the system must identify, contain, and, if possible, repair faults while providing timely notification to human operators.

Design of Embedded Real-Time Systems. Medical devices are embedded not only inside information networks but also inside human patients, whose critical life-functions they monitor and regulate. The design of medical devices is therefore more than an IT issue; it must also include the devices' interaction with patients and the environments and contexts in which they coexist. Thus we need a fundamental rethinking of medical-device design— toward a holistic approach that integrates functional, computational, and communication designs in the presence of uncertain patient models, in both normal and abnormal conditions.

Validation and Certification. Current design practice makes certification and validation an afterthought, at the end of the design cycle, when it is frequently too late to change design choices. As medical devices become more complex and more interconnected, it is becoming increasingly evident that certification should be incorporated in early design stages. Furthermore, certification and design frameworks are based on full systems, not components, resulting in time-consuming and expensive certification of large integrated systems, inefficient certification of incremental or evolutionary designs, and difficulties in maintaining or upgrading legacy systems.

New Research Directions

Despite the nationwide scale and heterogeneous nature of the R&D challenges, the following list of research directions will help us make significant progress toward realizing the outlined vision.

Infrastructure for Medical-Device Integration and Interoperation. The Electronic Health Records initiative needs to be safely and securely integrated with plug-and-play interoperable device networks. We could then fully realize the vision of actively using patient-specific information for optimum health delivery via interoperable medical devices. Interoperability has presented a major challenge to integrating medical devices from different manufacturers. It will require the development of standards and architectures not only for medical records but also for devices that actively use that information to monitor and regulate patients' medical conditions. Besides unique patient (record) identifiers, which must support the integration of devices from different manufacturers, standards must address data and communication formats as well as the contexts and environment assumptions in which the information will be interpreted and used.

Model-Based Development. The multifaceted nature of designing, implementing, and certifying medical devices requires holistic frameworks that are simultaneously based on models and components. Because of the strong coupling between device and patient, model- based frameworks that explicitly model devices' interaction and limitations with the environment and with the patient would lead to safer, higher-confidence devices and, ultimately, better health care.

Component-Based Design Frameworks. Component-based frameworks have been developed to facilitate the reuse of large and complex systems through the reuse of individually deployable and reusable components. Despite substantial progress in developing component-based frameworks for non-embedded software, such frameworks have rarely been applied to medical-device software and systems. An integrated approach that combines component-based and model-based development is an important research direction that can meet development and maintenance challenges of medical-device software and systems. Component-based development for both design and certification will dramatically affect the design and certification process: it will enable incremental yet certified compositions of certified components, allowing the safe and rapid reuse of legacy components (models, software, and algorithms). Our goal should be to develop frameworks in which certification is part of the design process rather than an afterthought. Component-based design should also support a variety of standards for communication and security.

Patient Modeling and Simulation. Medical devices face a unique challenge in model-based design, because of the scarcity of patient models and high-fidelity simulators for device design. As future devices adapt to patients, their medical conditions, and the environments they live in, it will be important to develop a variety of models and simulators for normal and abnormal patients in a variety of physical and environmental conditions. We must develop models and simulators at various levels of detail, ranging from coarse models for device design to high-fidelity simulators for model validation and virtual validation and testing.

Adaptive Patient-Specific Algorithms. Whereas medical devices are typically designed for groups of patients who have similar medical conditions, we could dramatically improve health care by making devices whose operation would adapt to a specific patient's specific medical condition. To achieve that, we need to develop algorithms for medical devices that are certifiably safe for large classes of patients and that can adapt to individual patients or to different environments that patients may be living in.

Requirement and Metrics for Certifiable Assurance and Safety. The development of rigorous requirements for clinical and design purposes, as well as metrics for certifiable assurance, are important research directions. Ideally, it should be possible to extract or convert natural-language clinical requirements to quantified engineering requirements. Such requirements make it possible to develop testing, validation, and analysis techniques with quantifiable guarantees for MDSS.

User-Centered Design. As medical devices permeate cross-sections of society and all educational and technical backgrounds, ergonomics and ease-of-use issues in human-device interfaces should become important factors in design. User-centered design, ergonomics, and ease-of-use issues in human-device interfaces should be considered throughout the design process. User and context modeling will result in better interaction between users and devices, minimize unsafe device operation, and result in graceful degradation of performance in the event of user or device failures.

Research Roadmap

Achieving this grand agenda is not simply a matter of time. It needs planning and support from government agencies. Here we offer a sequence for the most important components of a research roadmap that addresses the research challenges. Finally, this agenda has the potential to create a new scientific community and a new generation of scientists and engineers who integrate computer science, control theory, biomedical engineering, and medicine.

The proposed roadmap, which will dramatically affect medicine and health care, consists of three distinct phases.

Three-Year Roadmap

To develop a coherent body of methods and technologies that can meet the challenges of future MDSS, research needs are not just in information technology but in something that is much more multidisciplinary and involves significant computer science along with biomedical engineering, device manufacturing, and the medical-care process. In three years, we would like to see—

An initial set of publicly available open experimental platforms that contain design artifacts, including reference models and usage scenarios of different medical devices, so that researchers can obtain empirical feedback on their ideas about real-world systems

The development of standards for data, information, and communication to enable plug-andplay medical devices and to support interoperable device networks

An understanding of the approval process, along with the formalization of clinical and user- centered design requirements, and the development of quantifiable metrics for system assurance and certification

The formation of an R&D community for medical-device design to raise awareness across different subdisciplines and to foster collaborations between researchers, industry, health care providers, and government agencies

Five-Year Roadmap

For the slightly longer term, we would like to see short-term technologies enter clinical trials. Examples are standards-based compliance specification, verification, and validation technologies and processes for interoperability and QoS. In addition, we should focus on the theoretical and engineering foundations for system engineering aspects of medical infrastructures. In five years, we would like to see—

The integration of technologies for medical devices that have different QoS requirements into a network-centric system of systems, including management systems for medical information and networked devices in an operating room

A fundamental understanding of how to carry out the medical-practice-driven design of components and protocols so as to improve the safety of medical devices

A demonstration of the practicality of model-based frameworks for MDSS development and integration

The development of certification methods for individual components and networks of devices, and the development of an evidence-based, technology-aware certification process

Ten-Year Roadmap

Further out, we would like to see FDA-approved networked medical devices in wide use, with a medical infrastructure that supports the composition and integration of medical-device components while guaranteeing QoS, security and privacy, validation, and certification. In particular, the research and development of MDSS should culminate in—

The deployment of a fully integrated hospital intensive-care system using distributed monitoring, distributed control, and real-time wireless networks

The development of FDA-approved certification methods for medical-device software and systems and networked in-home patient monitoring and assistance

The availability of high-fidelity organ and patient models for design, testing, and validation and model-based frameworks that support component-based modeling, design, testing, and certification using patient models

DISTRIBUTED SENSING AND CONTROL IN NETWORKED MEDICAL-DEVICE SYSTEMS

Participants: Bruce H, Krogh (chair), Tarek F. Abdelzaher, Timothy Buchman, Rich Craft, Mike Eklund, Sandeep K. S. Gupta, Nagarajan Kandasamy, T. John Koo, Ronald

Marchessault, Tom Martin, Douglas Miller, Klara Nahrstedt, Tariq Samad, - Wei Zhao, George Fainekos (observer), Sebastian Fischmeister (observer)

Introduction

The networking of medical devices for distributed sensing and control occurs at many levels, ranging from dedicated networks of devices for individual patients to wireless networks for monitoring residents in long-term-care facilities. These networks may collect data for off-line analysis, generate alarms when critical conditions occur, or close feedback loops for the controlled delivery of drugs. Networks are increasingly being used to distribute stored medical information for remote diagnosis, such as picture archive and communication systems (PACS) that distribute x-rays and other images. In the future, wireless networks will supply distributed data acquisition and control for patients who are free to live relatively normal lives in their communities. Networking is the essential enabling technology for future advances in monitoring, diagnosis, treatment, and effective responses to acute conditions.

The growth of network applications for medical devices using current commercial off-the-shelf technologies (COTS) has been rapid. Development has been ad hoc, however, focusing on particular applications—with little standardization. Current COTS networks do not provide a sound basis for highly distributed medical-device systems that offer guarantees of security, privacy, robustness, interoperability, extensibility, mobility, and general patient safety. Research is needed to create medical-device networks that have such features, in order to improve health care in multiple dimensions and to enable the rapid dissemination of new sensing and control technologies as they become available. The following sections elaborate on these research needs and challenges.

What Can We Do Well?

Currently, data can be collected and sent to a variety of devices, such as—

Implantable devices, such as pacemakers, defibrillators, nerve sensors, and neurostimulators
Devices for patient monitoring, such as electrocardiogram, pulse oximetry, transcutaneous oxygen, electroencephalogram, pulmonary testing, and spirometry
Devices for point-of-care testing and monitoring in assisted-living environments

The use of existing COTS network technologies to collect data from such medical devices is growing. Networks are used to log data and provide real-time alarms to attending health care personnel for patients in intensive-care units. EKG monitors for multiple patients are networked to deliver information to a shared database. In assisted-living facilities, monitoring devices are networked in several ways, including wireless networks that monitor ambulatory patients.

Networking is also facilitating in-home health care. Many people have wireless devices that they can use to request immediate assistance in their homes. In-home monitoring systems regularly and automatically deliver data on blood pressure, heart rate, and glucose levels over phone lines to databases that physicians can access. Home monitoring systems are also available to send alarms for congestive heart failure to emergency response professionals.

In hospitals, raw sensor data is often transmitted over networks, using standards for laboratory information systems, with basic analysis to flag obvious outliers. Networks also play a significant role in emerging systems for therapy and surgery. For example, networks connect sensors, processors, and controllers in radiation therapy systems to perform real-time tumor tracking. Similarly, networks are being used as an alternative to dedicated point-to-point connections of devices in systems for telerobotic surgery.

Why Can't We Declare Victory?

Despite the successes of networking medical devices, they face significant barriers to realizing their full potential. COTS networking technology is typically optimized for bandwidth rather than time delay, making it difficult to optimize the performance of critical real-time feedback loops. For example, one system for the real-time tumor tracking of treatment beam control has to be operated in a degraded mode because its several networked components for signal processing and control provide no timing guarantees.

Also, current systems are fragmented and often incompatible. Although individual devices continue to become more sophisticated, they cannot "talk" to each other. For example, acute-care medicine (including ER, OR, ICU, radiology suites, and anesthesia), which of all medical areas is the best served by networked monitoring, is only now starting to see some data continuity. The lack of standards prevents the integration of information needed to provide the physiological basis for interpreting and acting on the increase in sensing modalities.

Another shortcoming of current networked systems is a lack of significant processing of information. It has been noted that medical systems are now awash in data but are information poor. Monitoring systems deliver data, but human experts need to interpret the data. When interpretation is attempted, it needs to be carefully evaluated. For example, in ICU monitoring systems, false alarms are far too frequent to rely on without extensive human intervention. The ability to glean useful information based on the fusion of data from multiple sources on a network is virtually nonexistent.

The delivery of the correct information will be particularly important in telemedicine, where a network will provide the only direct, real-time information available to the human. Sensor fusion is also needed, to provide correct information to the computer that closes feedback loops. In robotic surgery, for example, the human surgeon must receive haptic feedback, and correct information must be provided to the robotic surgical assistant, which needs precise knowledge of the location and type of tissue in the workspace.

Medical systems must also become more intelligent in the ways they interact with human users. Current devices and systems merely respond to operator inputs in a deterministic way. Beyond simple limit checking, they have little internal monitoring or analysis of the commands they receive. Given the diversity of training and skills of the individuals who will interact with future medical systems, it is important to consider all aspects of the human factors. As medical systems become more sophisticated and automated, they will need the ability to identify the level of knowledge and skill of the operator—and to respond appropriately. For example, when a system receives inappropriate sequences of commands that could be detrimental to the patient, the system should respond by maintaining a safe operating condition and supplying clarifying information to address the possibility of confusion by the user. Self-monitoring networked devices could adapt to changes in the user over time. As a patient ages, for example, a device might become easier to use by providing more detailed and thorough instructions.

Specific R&D Challenges

For our discussion, we will divide R&D challenges into two categories: component level and system level.

Component Level

The challenges of interoperability and compatibility are perhaps the most important to address immediately so as to facilitate the development of networked medical devices. We need to create standards, based on sound computational principals, with clear semantics. We need to develop middleware, in order to provide standard interfaces between medical devices and networks. That will make it possible to integrate components at the time of use rather than at the time of design.

Advances are needed in embedded-systems technology so that quality-of-service (QoS) guarantees at the component level can guarantee performance at the system level. The relative importance of security, privacy, robustness, interoperability, extensibility, mobility, and general patient safety must be evaluated carefully. Those issues need to be addressed by heterogeneous teams of computer scientists and health care professionals. The undertaking should begin with the establishment of a clear, mutually understood, shared vocabulary.

Devices must operate safely under all possible fault conditions and must provide appropriate information under all conditions. For example, when devices become disconnected from a network, caregivers often conclude that the devices are faulty. Devices and the network infrastructure must be designed so that in such situations, correct default values are delivered to the system. And the individual devices need to have mechanisms that indicate their states when they are not connected to the network.

Model-based design is a significant trend that facilitates the complete development process for embedded systems—from the capturing of requirements to implementation and deployment. The model-based approach builds partly on precise, formal descriptions that define the embedded system in relation to the domain in which it will apply. The medical domain requires a new formal language to support dialog among clinicians, physiologists, and device designers for the development of medical devices that are founded on a common, integrated framework. This formalization of the domain will also lead to new methods of component-level certification for safety-critical software.

A new model-based approach to the design of medical devices will also make it possible to address the many critical constraints in medicine, including form factor, power limitations, and usability. From an information technology perspective, formalizing the requirements and features of networked medical devices will make it possible to leverage emerging technologies much more quickly than we can today. Such technologies include smart sensors, digital video processing, and new methods of power management, such as harvesting energy from the environment.

Systems Level

Connecting components into workable, effective medical systems requires advances in system integration technologies. Distributed sensing and control need standards and architectures that make it possible to create networks of diverse medical devices and medical information systems.

The support of real-time critical services must be based on models of end-to-end service that account for the details of sophisticated interconnection technologies.

System-level power management will be a necessary part of the monitoring and control of medical devices for patients beyond the walls of hospitals and health care institutions. Accomplishing the goal will require a full systems engineering approach—one that identifies the parts of the system that must be reengineered to provide the needed QoS for the complex systems of systems that arise in distributed medical monitoring and control.

Research is also needed in medical information and algorithms. Effective systems for model- based monitoring and control must include algorithms for learning and adaptation that adjust parameters appropriately for each patient. Data manipulation schemes must be developed to support the integration of electronic health records (EHR) with information from medical monitoring systems and clinical decision-support systems. Given the rate of innovation in medicine, it is also essential that information management systems are designed to be extensible, so that new types of information can be integrated easily and immediately without requiring any amount of redesign.

System-level research must regard information security and privacy as issues of primary concern. Incorporating support for privacy techniques—such as selective disclosure, auditing the auditors, and encrypted searches—are essential in networked medical systems, because of the safety-critical and personal nature of information. For security and privacy, system-level information authentication schemes need to be developed.

Effective medical monitoring and control can be done at the system level only by drawing on different sources of information to make correct decisions. Besides developing new algorithms to perform sensor fusion for medical applications, research is needed to determine how the diverse sources of information can be used to validate data and even to calibrate distributed equipment. For long-term monitoring, device maintenance can be scheduled by the integrated information system.

Model-based development can help address one of the major human-factor issues: training. Models used for component-level design and system integration could become the basis of sophisticated simulation-based training systems. The use of simulators for training, which is standard in other areas involving complex technologies—such as aircraft and power systems— could reduce the cost of training and could raise the comfort level and acceptance of new networked technologies in medicine.

Human factors also play an important role in the potential for networked monitoring and control in medicine. Systems must be ergonomic, having human-machine interfaces that encourage acceptance by patients and caregivers and that consider the skill sets of the end users. Local control loops and control over networks need to take into account the full implications of possible human intervention. It is also important that systems be designed so as to enhance the capability of medical professionals to provide high-quality care—and not convey the message that the networked information system is attempting to remove the human from the loop.

New methods are also needed to enhance the safety of medical systems. When abnormal conditions occur, a system should provide timely notification to operators, and performance should degrade gracefully rather than abruptly, especially in life-sustaining medical equipment. This capability requires modeling and implementation technologies that naturally support self- monitoring and prioritized functionality, along with real-time response.

To address the several issues described above, new metrics must be developed to measure the capabilities of systems in multiple dimensions and to evaluate the trade-offs between them. These metrics should deal with the distinctive features of the medical domain, including the diversity of the patient population, the complexities of the conditions being monitored and controlled, and variation in the knowledge and skills of the end-user community. These metrics could support run-time operation strategies as well as design-time evaluation.

Research Strategies and Roadmap

From the discussion above, the following four themes emerge as specifically IT-related research needs:

> ***Standards and Architectures***. True interoperability and extensibility for networked medical systems will be possible only when widely accepted standards are embraced. Moreover, an effective infrastructure to support such systems should be built on open-source middleware for distributed systems designed specifically for medical applications.
>
> ***Formal Models.*** English-language descriptions of requirements and specifications are too ambiguous for developing networked medical systems. We need a language with formal precision that will eliminate any possibilities for confusion that could arise when clinicians, physiologists, engineers, computer scientists, and others work together to develop safety- critical systems. These formal models can become the basis for the verification and validation of networked medical systems.
>
> ***Model-Based Design Tools.*** At both the component and the system levels, effective designs will need model-based tools. Models for the distributed monitoring and control of medical applications must be developed with representations that support the needs of domain experts as well as methods for analysis and implementation.
>
> ***Test Beds.*** We need prototype problems that can serve as test beds for pre-competitive research. Problems from the device level to the system level—including critical features of users (clinicians) and patients—must be defined clearly, and examples must bc disseminated widely, so that IT specialists can become fully engaged in developing the fundamental technologies.

To create a clear vision for research, we propose a roadmap, with milestones that stretch well beyond the capabilities of current systems. Those milestones, defined in terms of the capabilities of prototype systems, provide a basis for discussion among the many stakeholders in the medical and IT communities.

Three-Year Milestone: *A deployed networked sensing and control system on a mobile distributed population with more than 1,000 nodes.* In this system, ambulatory patients will be instrumented with continuous EKG tracers and pulse oximeters, and local closed-loop oxygen bottle control will be implemented. Features to be demonstrated include—

End-to-end QoS design
Remote processing of data
Integration with the EHR system
Multivendor support with autoconfiguration ("plug and play")
Smart sensors and smart alarms (few false alarms)

Five-Year Milestone: *Configurable communication, sensing, and control for emergency-room (ER) and geriatric care.* This milestone will have higher bandwidth and more sensing modalities than the three-year milestone. It will introduce additional sensing and control for glucose and insulin. Model-based development tools will provide simulation-based tools for medical training.

This system will feature—

Point-to-point communication
Patient localization
Service discovery and negotiation within the network
Secure network reprogramming
Service virtualization
Enhanced distributed control of local feedback loops

Seven-Year Milestone: *Integrated portable preoperative and postoperative monitoring for civilian and combat scenarios.* This wide-area distributed system will include advanced capabilities such as—

Ambulatory ultrasound monitoring
Blood vessel graft monitoring
Remote radiologic evaluation

The system will provide the possibility of real-time dosage adjustment based on remote monitoring and diagnosis. The network will operate in an ad hoc mobile environment with a very high bandwidth and guaranteed QoS for time-critical features. Feedback loops will be closed both locally and remotely, using patient-specific models. Treatment planning will be semiautonomous, and information fusion will provide robust smart alarms.

Ten-Year Milestone: The technology roadmap presented here culminates in the following two demonstrations comprising the ten-year milestone.

A fully integrated hospital acute-care system using distributed monitoring and control

A demonstration of the impact of long-term deployment of networked in-home patient monitoring and dosage control

These two systems will incorporate all of the advances advocated for distributed sensing and control of networked medical devices, including the application of extensible prototype standards and architectures for future development. The systems will also demonstrate the application of formal models and model-based design tools.

Concluding Remarks

Medical diagnosis and treatment draw on multiple sources of data, ranging from patient records to data supplied by real-time monitors. Current networking technologies have the bandwidth to acquire and deliver the data, but there are many barriers to realizing distributed sensing and control in networked medical-device systems. The barriers include a lack of adequate standards, a lack of effective algorithms to generate important information from the many crucial sources of data, and the unavailability of test data and nonproprietary experimental systems for research and development. The proposed roadmap provides a set of specific aggressive milestones that will drive the basic research and development to realize truly intelligent distributed medical systems in the next ten years.

Medical Infrastructure

Participants: Lui Sha (chair), Ashok Agrawala, Chris Gill, Julian Goldman, Jennifer Hou, David R. Jones, Soon Ju Kang, Raj Rajkumar, Majid Sarrafzadeh, Sang Son, Jack Stankovic, Simon Szykman, Russell Taylor, Taieb Znati, Madhukar Anand (recorder)

Introduction

Networks of networked embedded systems create many new possibilities and challenges. The next generation of medical systems is envisioned to be a ubiquitous network of networked systems for secure, reliable, privacy-preserving, and cost-effective personalized high-quality health care. It will be a network that improves the quality of life.

The current system consists of many standalone devices. Even if they are networked, most devices function on their own. For example, a nurse is alerted when a patient's electrocardiogram (EKG) becomes seriously abnormal. Hurrying to the patient's room, however, the nurse might see a contagious-disease warning sign at the entrance and realize that she or he should have put on protective clothing before entering. Memory lapses are common under stress.

In the future, all relevant information—such as the contagious-disease warning and special equipment needs—will be displayed along with the alerts. Thus the EKG machine will no longer be a standalone device and will become an integral part of a network: a network of medical devices and patient management. Patients' medical records and their current state, no matter where they are generated or collected, will be integrated, filtered, and delivered in real time to where they are needed.

During a surgical operation, context information—such as sensitivities to certain drugs—will be automatically routed to relevant devices, such as infusion pumps, to support personalized care and safety management. How the patient's vital signs are reacting to medications and surgical procedures will be correlated to streams of imagery data, selected and displayed in real time and tailored to the needs of medical personnel, such as surgeons, nurses, anesthetists, and anesthesiologists. For some particularly difficult stage in an unusual operation, an expert surgeon could remotely carry out the key steps, using remote displays and a robot-assisted surgical machine, avoiding the need to fly across the country to perform, say, 15 minutes of work. Furthermore, data recording will be integrated with storage management so that surgeons can review operations and key findings for longitudinal studies of the efficacy of drugs and operational procedures.

Networks of networked medical devices hold many promises. Besides enhanced operational capabilities derived from integrated devices and medical-information systems, they allow flexible configuration and deployment, and the collection of more accurate and representative data from natural settings for longitudinal studies to support improved health management. They also raise many challenges.

From the perspective of infrastructure technologies (other than networking technologies for connectivity), much remains to be done.

What Can We Do Well?

Over the past decade, and especially since the development of the World Wide Web, many technologies have been developed to support distributed computing systems. The emergence of middleware enables and simplifies the integration of components developed by multiple technologies: It provides a consistent set of higher-level network-oriented abstractions that are much closer to application requirements than what is done now. That simplifies the development of distributed and embedded systems. Middleware also provides a wide array of common services—such as name services, logging, and security—that have proved necessary to operate effectively in a networked environment. Successful commercial middleware includes J2EE, CORBA, and .NET. They are the foundation on which many Web-based applications are built.

This raises an interesting question: why don't we use these commercially available technologies to network systems?

Why Can't We Declare Victory?

Current medical devices are mostly standalone subsystems that have proprietary designs. Medical workers often must manually enter data and transfer it between machines. Sometimes, they need to set devices manually, so as to emulate the interlock needed between different devices and actions. So if a patient has medication Y, the limits of delivery X in an infusion pump need to be adjusted to Z. Medical workers also need to mentally correlate many paper records and screen displays from various diagnostic and monitoring machines. The process is time consuming, burdensome, and error prone.

The commercial middleware cited above does help, but it is limited to information management for medical records. Many record formats for patient identification depend on particular designs that their manufacturers provide. They cannot be extracted from their native environments and put into a universal patient identification database. Once we develop a common patient ID standard and migration process, we can readily apply commercial distributed-computing technologies.

Beyond record management, the primary two challenges in the development of integrated medical systems are safety and liability. They are intertwined. Many medication devices are safety critical. The FDA approves each device separately, in a specific application context. If we connect them and something goes wrong, who is responsible? Technically, this is a safety question. In the new interactive environment, how is safety specified? Is it specified correctly? Is it implemented correctly and does it perform as specified? Is there a proper training process for users? Do medical personnel use it correctly?

What makes these questions impossible to answer is that current commercial infrastructure software assumes absolutely no liability and has many known and unknown bugs. The development of a certifiably safe infrastructure for networked systems of medical systems is a long-term R&D challenge that involves not only advanced technologies but also a legally sound certification process.

Before we can have a certifiably safe medical network infrastructure, safety-related actions should be limited to computer-aided actions that are closely supervised by medical personnel as an intermediate step in its evolution. Even with this modest goal, we still have a way to go, because the current distributed infrastructure is a best-effort system whose real-time reliability and security cannot be ensured.

In the following sections, we will take a more detailed look at each of the challenges.

Specific R&D Challenges

Designing for Certification

Many medical devices are safety critical and must be certified. At present, the FDA approves medical devices. Certification is desirable but needs R&D to make it possible for medical-device software and systems. Thus, it is important to develop a standards-based infrastructure of certifiable networked medical devices so that we can reduce the costs of development, approval, and the deployment of new technologies and devices.

Certification cannot be an afterthought. We must develop technologies for the specification and the design of verifiable and certifiable medical devices. Certification includes devices' operational environments. In future integrated medical-device and medical-information systems, the application contexts might be quite dynamic. The development of technologies that can formally specify both application contexts and device behaviors is a major challenge for the vision of certifiable plug-and-play medical devices.

It will be vital that researchers work with medical and regulatory agencies to ensure compliance with safety requirements. In addition, they will need to work with the Institute of Electrical and Electronics Engineers (IEEE), the International Organization for Standardization (ISO), and other standard-setting entities to develop voluntary market-driven certification for (1) interoperability and compatibility standards and (2) quality-of-service (QoS) standards—such as real-time fault tolerance, privacy, and security.

Two challenges in this area are—

How to develop evidence-based safety certification technologies and processes, including technologies for specification and verification and validation

How to develop open-standard-based compliance specification, verification and validation technologies, and processes for interoperability and QoS properties

Quality of Service

End-to-end QoS is an important concern in the operation of medical devices. This section discusses key QoS attributes.

Managing Safety and Criticality

From operating room to enterprise system, different devices and subnetworks have different levels of clinical criticality. Data streams with different time sensitivities and criticality levels may share many resources of the hardware and software infrastructure. How to maintain safety in an integrated system is a major challenge that consists of many research issues:

How to develop a safety interlock for the operation of interacting devices

How to manage the flows of data streams that have different criticality on the same network

How to mediate and manage the interactions of devices that have different criticality.

How to authorize and authenticate. Who can talk to whom?

How to support the fail-safe operation of individual devices

How to ensure that erroneous data is contained and does not cascade

How to specify, design, and verify the safety and efficacy of networked medical systems in the presence of device hardware failures and software errors

Security and Privacy

Medical systems pose new challenges in security and privacy. For example, a patient may need to upgrade software that detects pacemaker arrhythmias using EMF (electric and magnetic fields)–based methods but that is impervious to EMF-based attacks. Emergency personnel may need to access private data on demand anywhere and anytime, especially in wireless environments. We need a better understanding of requirements for security and privacy in medical systems. These are some key aspects of that understanding:

How to develop a new model of security and privacy tailored to medical needs
How to develop a modular and flexible architecture that incorporates and evolves technologies for security and privacy
How to develop cost-effective solutions appropriate to the medical environment

Interoperability

Interoperability has been a major challenge in integrating medical devices from different manufacturers. When a device uses data supplied by other devices, what is involved is not only the format of the data but also the context in which to interpret the data. For example, is the blood pressure measured when the patient wakes up in the morning but is still in bed—or after a workout, or after taking medication? Here are important interoperability challenges:

How to specify the interface both for the format of medical data and for context information needed to interpret the data
How to specify, design, and verify the properties and compliance of interoperable hardware and software interfaces that go beyond the data format
How to develop a standard of unique patient (record) identifiers to support the integration of devices from different manufacturers
How to represent environmental assumptions implicitly embedded in code and make them machine checkable and user friendly
How to support the evolution of technologies and maintain interoperability between old and new devices

Real-Time and Scheduling Guarantees

Many medical devices operate in real time with different time constraints and different sensitivities to delays and jitters. In the envisioned network of networked medical devices, many types of real-time and non-real-time data traffic will share the same computing and communication resources. How to ensure the proper scheduling of real-time traffic is an important concern, and here are some of the challenges:

What should be the policies of resource allocation and scheduling that ensure predictable end-to-end timing constraints and interoperability
How to provide time-zone abstractions that can support monitoring and control loops that have differing time constraints, such as 5 milliseconds, 10 milliseconds, and 100 milliseconds
How to support consistent views and actions between distributed and collaborating medical devices within given timing constraints
When network equipment fails and a system is overloaded, how to ensure that deadlines for critical real-time data streams are met

Medical Information Management

Integrating the operation of medical devices with nationwide medical-information management will give us a better understanding of the effectiveness of medical procedures and provide the right context for treating patients. We need to build in support for integrated medical-information management:

How to perform the recording, correlation, and analysis of event sequences
How to provide real-time context awareness for the proper operation and management of medical devices and information
How to conduct real-time, context-aware alarm processing, filtering, and delivery (at present, false alarm rates are far too high)
How to integrate with enterprise systems to support record management and long-term studies
How to manage high-volume data intelligently. Aspects include—

- User-friendly real-time data collection, filtering, fusion, and delivery
- Support for storage networks and data mining
- Capability for TiVO replay during surgery
- Visualization of massive data sets

Wireless Medical Infrastructure

Wireless networking is an important enabling technology. To provide secure and reliable real- time communication, however, we face many challenges, including—

How to exploit ultra-wideband (UWB) technologies
How to improve interoperability and protect against interference
How to improve security, reliability, and schedulability
How to support mobility, including programming abstractions that manage mobility
How to integrate with the wired infrastructure

Research Strategies and Roadmap

In developing a high-assurance medical infrastructure, the priority is to create a system-engineering framework that integrates component technologies with certification technologies. It will be a grave mistake to develop different technologies in isolation. Although it is not overly difficult to develop protocols for safety, security, and real-time reliability and privacy in isolation for particular application contexts, those protocols sometimes interfere with one another unexpectedly when they are used together in different contexts.

Three-Year Roadmap

To create a coherent body of technologies that are certifiably safe, we must first gain a deep understanding of the context of medical applications. It is difficult to develop effective technologies without knowing the constraints. Three years from now, we would like to see—

An initial set of publicly available model application problems that allow researchers to understand user requirements and to test their ideas
An initial suite of coherent QoS protocols designed and rigorously specified and verified for correctness and compatibility
An initial set of experimental prototypes demonstrating the feasibility of new QoS and wireless technologies

Five-Year Roadmap

We would like to see short-term technologies enter clinical trials. Examples are standards-based compliance specification, verification, and validation technologies and processes for interoperability and QoS. In addition, we should focus on the theoretical and engineering foundations for system engineering aspects of medical infrastructures. In five years, we would like to see—

Network timing abstraction methods that support monitoring and control loops with multiple timing constraints, ranging from 1 millisecond to seconds to minutes.

Integration technologies for medical devices that have different QoS requirements into a network-centric system of systems, including management systems for medical information and networked devices in an operating room

Fundamental understand on how to design protocols that make certification easier and how to develop an evidence-based, technology-aware certification process

Ten-Year Roadmap

In 10 years, we would like to see FDA-approved networked medical devices in wide use, with medical infrastructures supporting the composition and integration of medical-device components while guaranteeing QoS, security and privacy, validation and certification.

How to model and reason about the interactions between protocols for safety, interoperability, real time, reliability, security, and privacy

How to design protocols that are compatible rather than interfere with one another

An evidence-based and technology-aware certification process defined for approval of medical device software and systems by regulating agencies

PATIENT MODELING AND SIMULATION

Participants: Harvey Rubin (chair), Ruzena Bajcsy, Scott L. Bartow, Amit Bose, M. Cenk Cavusoglu, Robert C. Kircher, Douglas Rosendale, Charles Taylor, Russ Taylor, David Arney (recorder)

Introduction

Convincing successes in other fields—such as aerospace, chemical plants, and the automotive industry—confirm the value of modeling. Among the benefits we see are novel product developments, increased safety parameters, cost effectiveness in development phases, and ultimately a higher rate of regulatory approval.

Patient models exist and evolve over five levels of the spatial scale. At each scale, the models involve heterogeneous structures and physical processes, and each model evolves over time. On the atomic and molecular level—at the angstrom scale—the models are manifest in biochemical and genetic systems. At the next level, the cellular level, models are actively being generated and investigated. These two levels are integrated into models of organ structure and function. Organ models are then integrated into models of whole-body function. At the highest level, societal interactions are modeled, where the models must accommodate the uniqueness of each patient and also must permit the aggregation of populations.

In the medical-practice domain, we anticipate that high-level modeling will result in improved health care, with better outcomes and a higher quality of care. We also anticipate that modeling will provide better use of health care dollars, with improvements in prevention, intervention, and maximal value and utilization of the electronic health record (EHR).

In product development, an argument can be made that patient modeling is a highly efficient tool in developing devices. The reasons are multifold. Among them: human studies are expensive; and device manufacturers need models for sophisticated protocols and the effective execution of procedures, planning, monitoring, and control. Currently, however, the barriers to developing specific models are high.

In training and professional certification, patient modeling provides outstanding opportunities for patient education and guidance in clinical decision-making.

In research, patient modeling offers a rich investigative platform on which to develop a wide variety of tools and techniques.

What Can We Do Well?

Functions and operations that patient modeling communities do well are found at the ends of the modeling spectrum. For example, although many parameters in enzymatic reactions have yet to be determined, the mathematical modeling of enzyme reaction kinetics is well established. Even reactions that follow stochastic rules are tractable with high-performance computing.

Another advanced example of patient modeling is found in medical imaging. When used properly, imaging has clearly been shown to be clinically cost effective and to have positive measures of outcome. Examples include seizure focus ablation, arrhythmia focus ablation, image-guided biopsies, and radiation therapy mapping. Imaging is also an important component at the procedural level, providing training environments and programs that are otherwise unavailable, costly, or dangerous. Some systems are already in use, indicating the potential for commercial success.

Remarkable advances in patient modeling have been made over the past five years at the subcellular level. For example, transcriptional analyses of a wide variety of diseases have been enabled by the rapid accumulation of microarray data coupled with the explosion of genome sequencing data. More complete mapping of the metabolome in various normal and disease states is accumulating as well. These data have been complemented by new techniques in data mining, analysis, and integration. Finally, modeling of the epidemiology of disease is a mature discipline, with well-developed tools and algorithms.

Convincing preliminary data shows that physiology-based modeling is effective. The critical- care domain and the intraoperative domain are two areas in which physiologic modeling is widely used. These areas are driving the development of even more sophisticated modeling software and devices. It is anticipated that the home-care and institutional-care markets will be the next to rely heavily on sophisticated patient modeling software and devices.

Patient models are the focus of a number of national and international funding agencies. Large government-funded programs have begun to support the development of tools necessary for patient modeling, and some already exist. For example, the Physiome project and the DARPA BioComp program support development at the biochemical, genetic, and cellular levels. The ITK open-source NIH-funded image processing toolkit focuses on tools for modeling at the organ and whole-body levels.

Other government programs in this realm are NASA's "digital astronaut" project, which is in the planning stage, and DARPA's Virtual Soldier project.

Why Can't We Declare Victory?

Patient models involve heterogeneous structures—atoms, molecules, cells, organs individuals, societies—**and physical processes that evolve in time and space**, posing difficult computational problems. We will call this the *multiscale/multistructure* problem.

Patient models must be accessible to a wide variety of communities. Fully integrated models must be available to large and heterogeneous communities, including practitioners, investigators, device developers, and regulators. Those communities are not tightly integrated; they do not generally participate in the same meetings; they do not share journals; and they are spread across industry, government, and even different departments in academic centers. We will call this the *communication* problem.

Mechanisms need to be developed to share data, models, tools, and results. The interoperability of models and the maintenance of privacy are two of the most challenging problems facing the field. In addition, both commercial and academic institutional barriers limit the sharing of data and tools. In the academic domain, the reward systems of appointments and promotions continue to rely heavily on independent contributions to knowledge creation and communication (research and teaching), although a number of national initiatives, such as the NIH Roadmap, address this issue. Commercial success clearly depends on resolving the issues of sharing, interoperability, and privacy. We will call this the *interoperability* problem.

Ultimately any patient model—whether molecular or societal—**is an abstraction of the real situation.** Therefore it is imperative to understand the theoretical possibilities and limitations of each domain-specific abstraction. This is the *abstraction* problem.

Improved computational techniques for assessing clinically relevant variability in measurements are needed. This is the *variability* problem.

Experimental validation of models using ex-vivo and biomimetic materials and systems, animal models, and clinical data is needed. This is the *validation* problem.

Specific R&D Challenges

Besides the six challenges mentioned above, we face least two infrastructure challenges:

Patient models need ongoing research and support.
Issues of policy—privacy, security, and legal and regulatory issues—must be investigated and recommendations developed.

Research Strategies and Roadmap

We suggest that the six challenges be initially attacked in two groups of three and that the following strategies and roadmap be developed:

Multiscale/multistructure, data variation, and abstraction problems. These challenges have been recognized as important and to some extent are funded by a number of government research agencies, including NSF, NIH, and DARPA. We recommend that participants in the relevant programs at each agency meet as the focus of a working group in a national symposium to review progress and define future directions with high-confidence medical devices and systems.

Communication, interoperability, and validation problems. We recommend that these challenges be addressed by developing a series of demonstration cases. To build the foundation for an open-source environment that (1) addresses issues of ontology, (2) includes links to available models, data, and device sources, and (3) develops protocols for validation, we recommend the creation of a "Knowledge Portal," consisting of a human anatomical atlas and a protocol manual, over the next two to five years.

Extensive data for the atlas exists, and new data may be readily available. The Veterans Affairs system already employs computerized medical systems, so the VA may be an excellent source of new data. The atlas should combine information from multiple patients and generate a coordinate system to "place" each patient. It should be searchable and should be able to generate statistical analysis. Ideally, the atlas would then be used to help predict outcomes based on individual characteristics and statistical outcomes. The atlas could help device companies to project the range of scales and sizes necessary for clinically useful devices.

The protocol manual would consist of detailed written descriptions of specific interventions, along with metrics to evaluate each intervention.

Three-Year Roadmap

Develop common ontologies:

Descriptions of blood vessel branching for predicting cardiovascular surgery outcomes
Descriptions of activities of daily living for safe performance in the home by the elderly

Five-Year Roadmap

Develop statistical and analytical tools to analyze "on the fly" randomized trials

Develop risk analysis tools that link procedures to outcomes

Develop statistical methods for characterizing variability, abnormality, and anatomical variance

Build multidisciplinary academic and industry teams for the production of high-confidence medical devices that will develop work plans; prioritize specific models; carry out preclinical and clinical trials to validate models and publish results of those studies; support the FDA approval process for the model and for medical-device validation; and maintain the model and support device manufacturers that use the model for FDA submissions

Although the above seem like complicated tasks, there is an existing example. The SRI/Stanford consortium consists of seven medical-device manufacturers to develop a model of a femoral artery stent. The consortium does data acquisition and modeling, and publishes the work, and the work product can be used for certification. Companies buy in and get prepublication data.

We recommend that the FDA, NSF, NIH, and NIST encourage public-private partnerships among academia, industry, and government.

Funding, privacy, security, and legal and regulatory issues are high-level, cross-cutting issues for the entire HCMDSS community. They should be addressed by an executive committee with representatives of academia, federal funding and regulatory agencies, and industry.

Concluding Remarks

Successful patient modeling will require the solution to a massive problem of information fusion and analysis. But the payoff to solving the problem is enormous. It will lead to better patient care at every level: better clinical results, better disease prevention, and, in principle, better use of costly medical interventions and potentially scarce resources. Fortunately, interest in the problem is intense across a wide range of biomedical, commercial, patient advocate, and regulatory communities. The challenge now is to integrate and channel that interest so that each community can contribute to the solution, recognizing that there is new knowledge to be generated, communicated, and implemented—knowledge that in the end could have a profound impact on the fabric of life represented in better personal and public health.

MEDICAL-DEVICE SOFTWARE DEVELOPMENT

Participants: Peter Lee (chair), Steve van Albert, Rajeev Alur, Douglas Barton, Ralph DePalma, Matthew Dwyer, Steven Getz, LeRoy Jones, Peter Kuzmak, Rami Melhem, Jens Palsberg, John Regehr, Victoria Rich, Michael Robkin, Gregg Rothermel, Vish Sankaran, Bow-Yaw Wang, Arvind Easwaran (recorder)

Introduction

Many medical devices are, essentially, embedded systems. As such, software is often a fundamental, albeit not always obvious, part of a device's functionality. This means that any safety and regulatory requirements for medical devices necessarily involve the verification and validation of software-based systems. Exactly how to accomplish that is a major question, particularly because devices and systems are becoming increasingly complicated and interconnected. We may already have reached the point where testing as the primary means to gain confidence in a system is impractical or ineffective.

Further, the lack of uniform standards in the engineering of medical-device software leads to many deficiencies, such as the lack of precise system specifications. Both lacks inhibit even the best testing approaches and make it difficult for domain experts (cardiologists, neurosurgeons, and so forth) to ascertain whether a device will perform appropriately—even if it has been thoroughly tested. The lack of standards goes beyond software engineering practices and development technologies. Although the physician who performs an operation must be licensed, the developers who create the software used in the devices have no licensing requirements. Thus it is especially important that designs and software both be subjected to rigorous analysis. Such analysis is fundamental to effective and efficient testing, the analysis of systems-of-systems, and the determination and mitigation of risk.

In today's medical-device industry, embedded software and applications are often designed and developed by medical specialists—not by experienced software engineers. Although medical specialists are sometimes effective and experienced programmers, they often lack the software design expertise that has been developed in software engineering over the past 40 years. Typically, shortcomings in software analysis and design lead to rigid software and nonstandard platforms that are not resilient to change. The lack of resilience ultimately reduces the operational life of the underlying applications.

Along with the software-quality issue, research evidence suggests that the "frequency and consequences of medical device use errors far exceed those arising from device failures" . This in turn suggests that techniques for *user-centered design* have not yet made a significant impact on medical-device design. Surveys reveal that medical-device manufacturers give variable attention to usability issues in device design. Also, modern medical practice continues to see dramatic increases in the already enormous amount of knowledge that clinicians must absorb and use. Medical devices often demand detailed knowledge of increasingly sophisticated and often fragile science and engineering. The trend reduces the probability that clinicians will understand the inner workings and essential mental models that underlie the technologies used in complex medical devices.

What Can We Do Well?

Recent years have ushered in many improvements in the technology and processes of software development. Even relatively simple tools and platforms, such as modern IDEs (integrated development environments), promote certain best practices (such as source revision controls) and are suitable for medical devices and systems.

Increasingly, manufacturers worldwide have adopted disciplined processes—such as those offered by the Capability Maturity Model Integration (CMMI) project—to help improve, assess, and sustain the quality of their products, along with their engineering, management, and methods of quality assurance. Those advances can have a great impact on the quality of medical devices, although they are not sufficient. Further research advances are necessary.

Medical Devices vs. Avionics Systems

A natural question is the extent to which the standards and practices used in avionics systems apply to software for medical devices. Although the two domains share the need for safety- critical software, their standards and practices have large differences. Perhaps the most striking is the almost complete lack of regard, in the medical-device software domain, for the specification of requirements. Those in the medical-device community often say, in essence, "We don't need requirements in developing medical devices."

Although such statements may seem startling, business models and incentives for medical devices lead to the development of highly proprietary technologies. This decreases the interaction among development teams and diminishes the perceived value, at least in the short term, of specifying requirements. It also presents a significant barrier to academic researchers' participation in medical-device technology—in sharp contrast to their participation in avionics.

Other technical metrics, such as availability and mean time to failure, also seem to be largely absent or appear only in diminished form in the development of medical-device software.

Culturally, the sense is that medicine is a "people-intensive" activity that necessarily has highly complex and individually tailored workflows. Although software is a critical enabler of those workflows, it is often viewed as a minor contributor to failures in the system, failures that can happen in many ways. So although information technology is a key enabler to lowering the cost and improving the quality of patient care, the software quality itself is not perceived to be, and in fact may not be, the single most critical issue.

It is unclear whether differences between avionics and medical-device software will continue to be significant. The development of each medical device as a separate "stovepipe" seems untenable for the future. Thus we anticipate that the development of medical devices will use practices much more familiar to the safety-critical software community, particularly as medical- device systems are used more and more in closed-loop situations—in which medical-device systems adapt to changes in patients' conditions without caregiver intervention.

Why Can't We Declare Victory?

The current state of the practice in medical-device software has several key problem areas. These are the most critical:

Poor Quality of Software and Software Architectures

The development of complex safety-critical software is the subject of much research in the computer science and software engineering communities. Even so, numerous IT-based medical systems have clearly identified faults that can be addressed without any advances in research. In some cases, easy technical solutions exist, but other barriers (usually nontechnical) prevent their application. Often those barriers involve the lack of standards, of interoperability, and of metrics in the field. Issues with legacy systems also hamper progress.

One system, for example, has a problem in which a Web form for one patient was automatically—and incorrectly—filled in with information for a different patient, most likely because of an interaction with "cookies" in the Web interface. In other cases, specific networking failures arise.

In still other cases, the faults lie in poor technical standards for interfaces and architectures. For example, the bar-coding system of the Bar Code Medication Administration (BCMA) lacks a uniform standard across blood suppliers. Furthermore, the bar-code tags themselves are physically unreliable. Those problems, coupled with faulty or incompatible bar-code readers, have led directly to patient deaths.

As yet another example, the identification system of the Digital Imaging and Communications in Medicine standard Health Level 7 (DICOM/HL7) is neither standardized in the industry nor properly implemented in deployed devices. This has led directly to the loss of medical records.

Some of those problems have immediate technical solutions that repair the faults and defects. But because they are legacy systems, applying the technical solutions poses many practical difficulties, even if the device manufacturers are made aware of the solutions. Furthermore, the market may or may not offer incentives to apply the solutions.

And so in each case, we have situations where specific algorithms and technical solutions may be known to the research community. How to apply them in the real world is a major question.

Feature Creep

Industry perceives that the market demands more and more features. This "feature creep" not only increases risk and complicates use but also leads to software interactions that are hard to specify and even harder to analyze. The result is that no one, not even the developers, understands how the systems behave.

Even in the research community, the value of testing and techniques for validation in the face of new features is poorly understood. Furthermore, developers lack metrics for reliability and usability, making it impossible to assess the costs and benefits of various validation approaches.

Usability Problems

Workflows and operations have become overly complicated because of the proliferation of devices and technologies. That proliferation has provided clear benefits to the quality and cost of patient care. But it can introduce significant and often unnecessary complications to hospital procedures. And it can lead to situations that are confusing to caregivers (such as task overload) and unacceptably perilous to patients.

Practitioners describe being on a "gadget treadmill," with constantly changing workflows and increasing distractions in the operating room. Some practitioners report difficulty knowing whether the operating room has been fully "switched on." In one OR, a nurse had the responsibility of making sure that the room was ready to go and that the operation could proceed, but the nurse was so focused on entering data that the main procedure was almost an afterthought! Such intensive distraction necessarily puts some patients in peril.

Beyond having to understand how to operate numerous devices, we see reported issues with version skew—situations where a device has two, three, or even more versions, whose interactions cause a system or network failure. Finally, when something fails, medical devices often have no audit capability, or "black box," that permits a post-mortem analysis of the failures.

Lack of Knowledge Sharing

"Knowledge saves lives" is a clear refrain in the medical community. Data can be transformed into information, and information into knowledge. IT is thus a key enabler, because even simple advances such as faster data entry can have a measurable impact on the number of lives saved. The sharing of information is hampered by the lack of interoperability standards and technologies and by confusion over privacy regulations, specifically the Health Insurance Portability and Accountability Act (HIPAA).

Aggravating the problem is the medical-device industry's proprietary nature. Each medical device or system is developed largely on its own, with little regard to the sharing of critical information across systems. Manufacturers seem to have clear commercial incentives *against* standardization, which presents yet another barrier to information sharing.

Lack of a Systems Engineering Perspective

Integrating technology into the clinical environment—which includes practitioners, workflows, and specific devices—often lacks a holistic, systems perspective. Many medical devices are designed, developed, and marketed largely as individual systems or gadgets. Device integration, interoperability, and safety features are not considered during development, acquisition, or deployment.

The situation is not unique to medical devices. In both research and development, the tendency is to look at systems in isolation, ignoring how well they will work in a larger setting. Workflow issues, including people and clinical procedures, could be reengineered to make safer and more optimum use of some technologies, but that is rarely considered.

The lack of a systems perspective results not only in safety problems but also in lost opportunities for exploiting advances in information technology. One issue that is in dire need of progress and for which there are exemplars in other industries is version skew. The automotive industry, for example, uses analysis and modeling tools that help manage version skew, but similar tools have not been widely adopted by the medical-device industry.

Specific R&D Challenges

Medical and assistive devices must be dependable. Dependable devices work as intended, are highly available even when not well maintained, and do no harm when they fail or are misused. Devices should also be customizable and easy to use, upgrade, and maintain.

Although those criteria apply to many domains of software application, we find that some research challenges and needs are either specific to medical devices or deserve additional emphasis compared with other domains. We summarize the challenges below.

Formal and Model-Based Analysis, Design, and Implementation

Methods of software engineering that are increasingly applied in other application domains go a long way toward improving the quality of software-centric systems. The methods range from relatively informal (though still disciplined) process models to rigorously formal methods based on mathematics and logic. One unifying theme is formal modeling.

At the relatively informal end of the spectrum, modeling languages such as the Unified Modeling Language (UML) and development methods such as Model-Driven Architecture (MDA) confer an important level of discipline and organization on the software design process. That discipline facilitates the early discovery of design problems and helps ensure that independently developed components work well together.

Although model-based approaches are normally applied to standard application software, experience shows that they also benefit embedded systems. But two features of medical systems—and of embedded systems in general—stand in the way of realizing the full potential of model-driven development. Correctness requirements for medical systems often include detailed operational requirements. Thus, commonly used modeling languages such as UML, which concentrate on a system's structural properties, fall short of the design needs. To make matters even more complex, medical devices work in complicated, dynamically changing environments. Without adequate modeling of the environment, it is impossible to make the model-based design of medical systems reliable. Also, the safety-critical nature of medical embedded devices requires a higher degree of validation than most software engineering processes provide.

Therefore, some amount of formal verification and validation needs to be at the core of modeling technology for medical software. We need modeling methods that naturally support operational specifications and enable rigorous verification; we need to incorporate those methods into existing design processes. The quest for such modeling techniques and practical formal methods will probably be the biggest challenge to design of software-based medical systems in the future.

Medical Practice–Driven Design and Validation

Like a sound foundation for integration, better tools and environments as described above can help us *build systems right.* Equally important is *to build the right system,* as pointed out by Wears and Berg in their March 2005 *Journal AMA* article "Computer Technology Still Waiting for Godot." The authors suggest that the root cause of errors such as the medication errors introduced by physician order-entry systems is that "the pattern of [IT] use is not tailored to the workers and their environment."

Although research has been performed on iatrogenic injuries (caused by a doctor or other caregiver), researchers rarely investigate medical errors involving poor device design. Besides patient injury, poor design causes other maladies, such as reductions in treatment efficiency and effectiveness, excessive training or maintenance costs, stress and confusion for users, and other attending complications. Any study based on patient harm, however, will vastly underestimate the systemic consequences and costs of poor integration and interface design. Specific usability challenges for overcoming those issues include the following:

> **Metrics for usability impact**. Studies have shown that, for example, the average software program has 40 design flaws that result in lost productivity. But little work

has been done on the impact of medical-device design. We need studies and data collection methods to better understand the impacts and costs of poor and suboptimal device design.

Capture and dissemination of usability guidelines. A wealth of literature exists on design principles for medical devices. But the knowledge is often relatively useless because it lacks information that attaches principles and guidelines to usability contexts. In addition, many guidelines are rarely updated. Given the fast pace of technological change, we need dynamic methods that capture and disseminate emerging knowledge.

User-centered design methods. Adhering to even the best usability guidelines and principles is not sufficient to guarantee appropriate device design. Diverse usability settings dictate that designers must work closely with users to match device design with specific practices and conditions of use. User-centered design methods have been created for design stages including requirements and inception, summative evaluation, end-user support, and post-release instrumentation and maintenance. What is missing is a means to unify those methods so as to better understand usability phenomena. In addition, existing user-centered techniques are not designed to address issues stemming from complex interacting systems (systems of systems) comprising users, devices, and use environments.

Diverse contexts of use. User interface design is difficult partly because interfaces are influenced by many situational variables. They include environmental context (such as offices visits, surgery, and emergency room), user populations (doctors, nurse practitioners, nurses, anesthesiologists), devices (internal, monitoring, analysis), interface type (device controls, screens, handhelds), and interaction type (selection sequences, parameterization, programming), to name a few. Design methods must therefore have the flexibility to accommodate the highly diverse and situation-dependent nature of interface design.

End-user programming and customization. Interface diversity is a direct reflection of the diversity of individuals and their medical conditions. Medical devices are designed with varying levels of end-user customization, from setting up parameters to tailoring environments involving forms of end-user programming that individualize therapies carried out by medical devices. As devices become more flexible, the potential for error increases. Medical-device interfaces must be designed to minimize and avoid life-threatening errors and parameter-setting combinations by, for example, detecting anomalies or outliers in parameters and making sure that programming directives do not break parameter invariants.

Clearly, we must adopt the user-centered approach, which calls for considering users (including caregivers, patients, and service personals) throughout the acquisition, design, implementation, and evaluation of requirements. Research is needed for user-centered design and quality assurance, including the creation of a library of user scenarios, user models, and their environments in the context of medical devices and systems based on real data. We also need standards similar to the International Standards Organization's ISO 13407 (User-Centered Design Process) to guide user-centered derivation of requirements and design and evaluation against the requirements.

Achieving User-Centered Designs for Medical Devices

Many techniques for modeling and analyzing user-interfaces are well known and have been investigated in various domains. But medical-device software is unique in many respects and brings concerns about safety and dependability that have not been adequately researched. We need empirical investigations so that we can better understand those specialized needs.

For example, it is important to ensure that at every step in a medical intervention, the supporting medical software reflects a valid state. At design time, standard medical procedures should be modeled in such a way that the use of the software is understood and documented. This may require development of workflows and use cases for medical procedures—and some efforts have been started in that direction. Later, preoperative models should be used in real time to confirm the steps necessary during the medical procedure. Monitoring approaches of this sort should also incorporate support for error-handling and fault tolerance. With solutions to these challenges, effectiveness of medical processes for common procedures can be evaluated and enhanced.

We also need state-based control standards, mechanisms, and diagnostic tools for medical software. Those items will help connect the actions in a medical operation with the corresponding actions of the supporting software. In addition, we need general validation approaches and real-time diagnostic tools to support preoperative and postoperative procedures. As a next step, general validation models should be investigated to validate medical processes during medical procedures.

Because context is vitally important to the development of high-confidence user interfaces, collecting and analyzing field data are crucial. Research is needed on technologies that capture not only data from laboratory studies, surveys, and interviews but also data from the field on operational software. Software instrumentation and profiling techniques, for example, could capture how users supply incorrect information and interact erroneously with devices.

Component-Based Design and System Integration

Contemporary software development emphasizes components that have clearly specified application programming interfaces (APIs). A static API for a software component such as a Java library class consists of all the (public) methods, along with the types of input parameters and returned values that the component supports. This promotes a clear separation between the specification of the component and its implementation. Such static APIs can be enforced using type systems of programming languages. But although type systems are indispensable, they offer only a partial solution to designing bug-free software, because they do not capture constraints on resources, real-time guarantees, and other quality-of-service aspects. Consequently, they offer little assistance in "system" integration. This is an important issue, not only for being able to derive system-level performance and correctness guarantees, but also for being able to assemble components cost-effectively.

The interface for a device that interacts with a patient must incorporate information about timing delays and continuous parameters such as threshold levels. Capturing the notion of quality-ofservice abstractly, and having mechanisms that can enforce the adherence to interfaces and that can check compatibility between interfaces, is already an emerging and challenging trend in research on embedded systems. The additional concerns with medical practice–driven design and formal analysis increase the need for advanced research. On the other hand, by identifying key component types relevant to medical devices, we open new opportunities to apply what is already known. Providing an impetus to the research community to understand and address the issue is a critical need.

Open-Research Test Beds

Today we have open-research platforms that provide highly effective support for the widespread dissemination of new technologies and even the development of classified applications. The platforms also provide test beds for collaborations involving both researchers and practitioners. One spectacular example is the Berkeley Motes system with the TinyOS operating system.

The medical-device community could benefit from the existence of such open-research platforms. They would enable academic researchers to become engaged in directly relevant problems while preserving the need for proprietary development by the industry. (TinyOS facilitates academic input even on government-classified technology, which is an example of what is possible.)

Taking steps to enable the creation of such test beds should be considered immediately.

Research Strategies and Roadmap

To achieve assurance guarantees for medical devices, we need a paradigm shift—one that includes a formal approach to design, implementation, and analysis. Model-based and formal methods have been successful in targeted applications such as microprocessor designs. Recently, formal verification tools have fully analyzed and verified a number of low-level (device-driver level) and embedded avionics applications. We believe that the same success is feasible in the domain of medical devices. Such an approach would comprise the following steps:

1. Define requirements of the system in a mathematically precise notation.
2. Design a high-level model of the control algorithm for the medical device.
3. Design a high-level model of the environment in which the device will operate.
4. Subject the device model, together with the environment model, to powerful analysis techniques, such as simulation, optimization, and verification.
5. Either generate code automatically from the device model or verify that hand-written code is consistent with the model.

Three-Year Roadmap

In view of these R&D challenges, it seems clear that research needs are not just in information technology but in something that is much more multidisciplinary and involves a systems approach. It includes significant computer science along with biomedical engineering, device manufacturing, and the care process.

Develop open, experimental platforms and standardized research data sets to foster collaboration between academic, industry, and industry

Extract models from clinicians and their workflows, analyze change effects, measure system performance, and so on, to support a systems engineering approach

Academia, industry, and the government should work together to address the technically straightforward, well-known deficiencies in today's medical IT systems. Specific examples are universally unique identifiers for medical-information objects and standardized bar-code technologies in blood bank applications and administration.

Five-Year Roadmap

In five years, it should be possible to perform experimental evaluations of the effectiveness of integrated systems:

Develop medical practice-driven design and validation, including metrics for usability evaluation and user-centered design methods

Device component-based designs and systems-integration-based formal models of medical devices, control algorithms, and workflows of medical practice

Create open-research test beds to disseminate new technologies and develop a set of applications

Ten Years

In ten years, we expect to have model-based techniques for producing complex integrated systems cost-effectively. The integrated systems will be subjected to quantifiable assurance measures that can be the basis for certification:

Develop model-based validation and certification of systems of medical device systems

Develop medical-device software and systems that can prevent misuses by caregivers, adapt to changing patient conditions, and can be safely used in closed-loop situations

FOUNDATIONS FOR INTEGRATING MEDICAL-DEVICE SYSTEMS AND MODELS

Participants: W. Rance Cleaveland II (chair), M. Brian Blake, Andrew Casertano, Sherman Eagles, Scott Henninger, David W. Hislop, Zachary Ives, Tomasz Petelenz, Jane W. S. Liu, Tom Martin, Gregory Sharp

Introduction

Medical technology is in the midst of a profound technological revolution. On the one hand, advances in computing have led to the development of novel diagnostic and therapeutic equipment and procedures, ranging from advanced imaging machines to minimally invasive surgical techniques and implantable heart devices. On the other hand, low-cost computing equipment and improved software have enabled the automation of many administrative aspects of health care, including hospital management and insurance-claim processing. The result has been operational efficiencies that open the door for the delivery of lower-cost, higher-quality care.

At the same time, the national dialog on health care continues to focus on the inexorable rise in costs and on concerns about the quality of care. The press lauds advances in standalone diagnostic and treatment systems—and rightly so. But systemic inefficiencies in health care delivery grossly inflate costs and contribute to avoidable medical errors that degrade patient care.

Those inefficiencies are primarily caused by a lack of mechanisms to create integrated medical systems that coordinate the collection of information and the delivery of medical services. The health of all Americans would benefit greatly from research into technologies that support the seamless and secure sharing of health information; enable the integration of hospital-based monitoring, diagnostic, and therapeutic devices; and provide capabilities for remote monitoring and the treatment of chronic disease.

The technical recommendations in this chapter derive from a core observation: The systems of medical devices needed to implement the data-sharing and distributed-care delivery described above are impossible to build in a cost-effective, timely manner. This stems largely from an ad hoc approach to designing, developing, and deploying such systems. There is a pressing need for well-understood models, theories, and tools for reasoning about medical-device interfaces, the composition and integration of systems from component devices, and systems of systems that support the predictive analysis of end-to-end system properties that are important to medical applications. Among those properties are—

Efficacy
Safety
Security
Privacy
Traceability
Confidence

What Can We Do Well?

This section characterizes the state of the art for medical-device and medical-system integration and modeling in terms of technologies used in three types of integration scenarios:

1. **Medical-information systems.** Such systems manage patient and caregiver information. The integration of such systems is intended to reduce the overhead and risks associated with information management.

2. **Point-of-care-based monitoring, diagnostic, and therapeutic device and systems.** These systems are typically overseen by medical experts. They are involved in the treatment of specific patient disorders. Integration issues include individual device design (Will a device perform according to requirements? Is a device easily and appropriately integratable with others) and system design (Will one device interfere with another? Can system behavior be easily inferred from the properties of an individual device?).

3. **Extramural monitoring, diagnostic, and therapeutic devices and systems.** These systems may be home based or implanted and thus are beyond the immediate control of medical personnel. Integration issues include the ones mentioned above for hospital-based systems. Other issues involve the delivery of information from these systems to caregivers in a manner that is timely and secure, and that respects privacy.

Communication Standards

Efforts to develop integration frameworks for medical devices and systems have focused on defining communication protocols and data-format standards for medical data. Some standards have focused on specific areas in medicine, a prominent example being the DICOM (Digital Imaging and Communications in Medicine) standard for medical imaging. DICOM defines a format for digital storage of images independent of imaging technology. It is in widespread use.

Other work has focused on issues related to the exchange of medical data among medical- information systems. For example, the mission of the Health Level 7 (HL7) standards organization is *"To provide standards for the exchange, management and integration of data that support clinical patient care and the management, delivery and evaluation of healthcare services. Specifically, to create flexible, cost effective approaches, standards, guidelines, methodologies, and related services for interoperability between healthcare information systems."* Standards developed by HL7 include the Version 2.5 Message Standard, which defines message formats and protocol standards governing patient control (admission, discharge), order entry (dietary, pharmaceutical), financial management, and the like. According to the HL7 Web site, Version 2.5 is the most widely implemented communication standard in the world. As part of the Version 3 Message Standard, HL7 has developed the Reference Information Model (RIM) for clinical and administrative health care data.

Other standards bodies have focused on point-of-care communication protocols. The IEEE 1073/ISO 11073 specification, for example, defines rules for connecting bedside devices so that that they can exchange data. The standard includes components for a variety of medical devices, such as respirators, defibrillators, and electrocardiographs. The IEEE 1073 Web site refers to 1073 as the basis for plug-and-play medical-device systems.

At present, no widespread standards exist for so-called extramural medical devices. The main reason is the relatively recent emergence of a wide variety of such devices that improvements in power consumption have enabled. Improved radio and infrared technology makes the communication of data from devices to external medical equipment feasible, but data standards have yet to be developed. Similarly, we know of no standards governing communication between point-of-care systems and medical-information systems. Although communication and data standards exist, the bulk of clinical and administrative information remains encoded either on paper or in proprietary computer systems.

Standards and Regulations for Medical-System Development

The development of medical devices and systems is a safety-critical undertaking. Faulty devices can endanger patients' well being and even lives. Most efforts aimed at improving the development of such devices have taken the form of standards and regulations governing best development practices.

The IEC 60601 family of standards is a case in point. The standards specify requirements for electrical medical devices (defined as those that have at most one connection to a power main and that transmit energy to a patient). They contain general information about electrical shock, radiation, and fire hazards as well as device-specific guidelines for electrical safety. The FDA recognizes IEC 60601 as a consensus standard and advises development organizations that adhering to the standard provides reasonable assurances of electrical safety.

The ISO 13485 standard for quality-management systems defines rules for assessing how robust a medical-device developer's quality-assurance processes are. The standard is an adaptation of ISO 9001 (a general quality-management system) for the medical industry and reflects the industry's considerable regulatory concerns. The revised Quality System Regulation (21 CFR 820, Oct. 7, 1996) (QSR) is also based on the ISO 9001 and ISO 13485 quality-system standards.

Other standards deal with risk management for medical devices. Emblematic is ISO 14971, which defines the components of a medical-device risk-management process, including policy development, training, and techniques such as Failure Mode and Effect Analysis (FMEA) and Fault-Tree Analysis (FTA), standard techniques for determining root causes of system failures.

Other governmental bodies have established regulatory frameworks to ensure medical-device quality. Of particular note are the Medical Device Directive (MDD, European directive 93/42/EEC), and guidelines for active implantable medical devices (90/3 85/EEC). These standards and regulations deal with individual medical devices, not systems of devices.

Design, Development, and Validation Technology for Software

As in other industries, the development of software for medical devices and systems remains largely a systems-based, standards-driven, document-intensive process. Standards such as those mentioned in the previous section are used to organize development organizations and to manage risk. The testing of device software is done primarily at the system level, using test benches containing hardware and software components. For radiological devices, "phantoms"—bags of fluid each about the size of humans, with sensors for measuring radiation exposure and the like—are used as mockups of human bodies to assess safety and performance.

Some organizations are beginning to use model-based design and development. Examples are use-case modeling of requirements for information systems and computer-assisted surgery, and state machines to model infusion pumps and implanted cardiac devices.

Such technologies are rarely mentioned in standards documents, which points to their immaturity in the medical arena.

Why Can't We Declare Victory?

The state of the art in medical-device and medical-system integration consists of two key components: low-level data-transfer protocols and standards, and standards and regulations specifying best practices for device development. Most medical information remains spread throughout hospitals and caregivers' offices and in insurance-company files. Patient bedsides consist of an array of devices connected, if at all, by cables that are easily disconnected and cause hazards. Operating rooms contain a hodgepodge of equipment and displays that can overwhelm medical personnel with data. Implanted devices suffer from recalls and operate in an information vacuum. After insurance paperwork, the first form a patient completes when visiting a doctor is still a medical history, which the patient may or may not recall. The transfer of data from the point of care to patient records still relies on human intervention.

Compare this situation with the following scenario. Everyone has an electronic health record (EHR) containing a complete account of his or her health history and current insurance information. That information can be queried by caregivers—no more haphazard history taking—and medical devices themselves, which could provide additional safety interlock features based on a patient's history. Bedside devices would communicate wirelessly—no cables—and could be configured to forward collected data automatically to a patient's medical record. Access to patient records would no longer be a bottleneck to consultations among caregivers. An operating room would feature a single integrated display for all equipment in the room, which would communicate with the display wirelessly—no cables to trip over—and would record information in "black boxes" for subsequent review of poor outcomes. Implanted devices and wearable monitoring equipment could record information in a patient's EHR, making it available for caregivers' review.

That vision represents a radical departure and entails significant investment in the research areas listed below. The benefits to human health, however, would offer a many-fold return on the investment.

Specific Research Challenges

Realizing the vision described above will require substantial research into technologies for medical-device and medical-system integration. The technologies are described below.

Electronic Health Records (EHR)

One backbone of the preceding vision is an accurate and complete electronic health record. Significant technical challenges confront the development of such a record, because of the extremely personal nature of individual health information and the many institutions that would need access to some, but not all, of the information. To be widely adopted, EHRs must be secure (to prevent unauthorized tampering) and provide privacy guarantees, so that control may be exercised over who has access to different components. In addition, EHRs must contain audit- trail mechanisms to record who has seen what. At the same time, those mechanisms must be minimally intrusive and must support incorporation of legacy health data, such as paper records.

Plug-and-Play Network Devices

Another enabling technology for the aforementioned vision is the development of plug-and-play networking technology for medical devices. Plug-and-play capability is needed to ease the setup of integrated point-of-care and extramural arrays of medical devices that communicate with a patient's electronic health record.

Devising the technology would require addressing concerns about privacy, security, safety, regulations, and technology. In hospital settings, for example, networks would form and reform frequently, as patients are admitted and discharged. Technology for the rapid formation of ad hoc networks needs developing. At the same time, authentication mechanisms would be needed to ensure that a device is on the correct network—and not, say, incorrectly attached to the one next door. Communication among devices would need to be made more secure than current wireless technology supports, and the problem of incorporating legacy devices must be addressed. Regulatory approaches ensuring the safety of open networks would need to be developed. Finally, for portable and implanted devices, plug-and-play technology would need to minimize power consumption, implying the need for low-power-consumption communication protocols.

Ergonomic and Ease-of-Use Issues in Human-Device Interfaces

The integration of devices in a care-giving setting requires careful attention to considerations of human factors—especially in extramural settings, where nonprofessionals would interact with devices. Issues of mode confusion and data fusion (combining data from various sources into a coherent form) will also need to be addressed, as point-of-care facilities become more complex and begin to resemble cockpits in airplanes.

Monitoring and Post-Intervention Analysis

In the integrated medical-device and medical-system setting considered here, faults and errors will occur: Devices will fail; caregivers will make mistakes; networks will crash. To cope with such problems, technologies must be developed for error handling, fault tolerance, fault diagnosis, and fault isolation in ad hoc wireless networks. "Black-box" standards—similar to those in aircraft—should be developed so that when systems do fail, lessons can be learned and responsibility assigned.

Component-Based Design and Validation

The technologies outlined in the previous sections will find use only as long as integrated systems of medical devices can be cost-effectively safe, robust, and secure. Current design and validation mechanisms for medical systems generally do not support open systems that share data while guaranteeing end-to-end privacy and security. Technologies for lifting reasoning about such properties from the single-device, single-component level to integrated component- based systems must be developed, most likely via notions of safety and security interfaces that would specify the safety and security properties that a component guarantees. Design patterns and service-oriented computing paradigms tailored for medical applications, with their specialized mix of security and privacy concerns, must also be built, and standardized modeling paradigms for open systems of communicating medical devices should be devised, so that "virtual" device networks can be built and simulated for validation purposes. Such simulation models would also be useful in training personnel.

To further support such virtual validation activities, accurate control-theoretic patient models must be developed so that medical-device model behavior can be simulated and assessed before trials on humans. Models of caregiver behavior should be developed for devices so that close- loop modeling of device, patient, and caregiver can be undertaken. Such simulations would yield useful information about likely caregiver errors in using devices, and that information could be used to improve user interfaces to devices and lower the likelihood of device misuse due to caregiver error. To guide subsequent system testing and risk analysis, we need to develop methods to quantify residual risk from virtual validation activities—how accurate are the data derived from simulations, and how can the analysis be used to focus efforts in subsequent clinical-trial testing? Strategies for in-vivo test planning based on virtual testing would open the door for additional efficiencies. Issues of data integrity and integration must also be studied. Efficient techniques for converting models into executing systems must be developed.

Open Experimental Platforms

The final component of an effective research program would be an open experimental platform for use by researchers investigating technologies to integrate medical systems and devices. Such a platform would contain design artifacts, including reference models and scenarios about the use of different medical devices, so that researchers could obtain empirical feedback on their ideas about real systems. An open experimental platform would be vital to the success of the research program, because concerns about intellectual property would otherwise preclude the sharing of device and system information.

Research Strategies and Roadmap

This section offers roadmaps for the research program outlined in the previous section.

Three-Year Roadmap

The goal in the first three years will be to begin developing conceptual frameworks for two core issues: the security and privacy of medical data.

> Reference models for privacy and security should be developed, with a view toward defining the stakeholders (such as patients, caregivers, insurance providers, and government) and the levels of access and control they have on patient information. Precise mechanisms for specifying the safety and security properties of medical software components must be developed, and use cases and reference models for standard medical devices such as infusion pumps, radiological devices, and cardiac devices must be elucidated. That software work will entail adapting software-design notations to medical purposes.

Control-theoretic models of human biological processes should be developed, and work on caregiver modeling initiated.

Five-Year Roadmap

The next phase of the research program will involve the development of tools and methods for technical support of the conceptual framework mentioned above. (The conceptual framework will continue to evolve.) Specifically—

Technologies will be developed for electronic health records that enforce the privacy and security policies for medical data.

Techniques for establishing end-to-end safety and security properties of systems based on component properties will be defined, and prototype automated tool support implemented.

Protocols for ad hoc secure networks of medical devices will also be defined, to ensure adherence to the security and privacy policies of medical data by collected data.

Virtual validation environments for medical devices, based on models of devices, human biology, and caregiver behavior, will be developed, and pilot studies will be conducted on the medical-device information contained in the developing open experimental platform.

Human-factors studies for medical-device interfaces will be initiated.

Service-oriented paradigms and design patterns for medical-device integration will be defined, and prototype tool support for the design of medical-device control systems begun.

Ten-Year Roadmap

The final phase of the research effort will focus on further developing the technologies and major case studies:

Implementations of electronic health records will be assessed empirically for utility and safety.

Improved control-theoretic models of human biological and physiological processes will enable a more thorough analysis of systems of medical devices, allowing the efficient development of multifunctional systems that enable the coordinated treatment of disorders with multiple causes (such as diabetes-induced heart disease).

Clinical trials will allow the quantification of residual risk in virtual, simulation-based validation approaches to medical-device systems, and as a result the virtual validation approaches will be refined.

Service-oriented design paradigms for medical systems will be codified, and design and validation tool support for them will be developed.

Secure, ad hoc networking protocols for medical applications will be implemented in both hardware and software, laying the basis for a commercial market for medical-device middleware.

Human-factors studies will feed into this work so that systems of medical devices can be assembled easily, and with user interfaces providing maximum support for caregivers and patients responsible for their use.

VERIFICATION, VALIDATION, AND CERTIFICATION

Participants: John Hatcliff (chair), Peter Coronado, Steve Dimmer, Jacob Flanz, Elsa L. Gunter, Mark P. Jones, Paul L. Jones, Brad Martin, Rosemary C. Polomano, Stacy Prowell, John Rushby, Rich Schrenker, Oleg Sokolsky, Aaron Evans (recorder)

Introduction

Verification and validation (V&V) tasks required for the approval of medical devices play a significant role in enabling the FDA to carry out its mandate of approving only "safe and effective" medical devices. Many industry observers believe that we are approaching the limits of reliable device V&V processes. As devices grow more and more complex and rely much more on embedded software to achieve critical functionality, existing methods are being challenged. The results: higher development costs for manufacturers, longer time to market, and increased chances of device failure—with associated recall or liability costs.

Today, V&V activities account for as much as half the cost of bringing devices to market. Moreover, it is important to consider the effectiveness and already high costs of verification, validation, and certification in the context of rapid advances in technology that have fundamentally changed the way many informational, financial, and scientific services are provided. Although technological advances have contributed to a steady increase in the quality of health care, and although V&V processes have for the most part been able to keep pace, we now seem to be on the cusp of the types of revolutionary changes in the domain of health care systems that have transformed other sectors of nation's infrastructure and economy.

For example, pervasive networking will enable the integration of national networks, regional health care centers, local hospitals and clinics, the offices of primary-care physicians, home computing, and body-area networks. And as generations of technology-savvy health care consumers enter retirement, they will embrace—and even demand—sophisticated home health care monitoring, treatment, and record systems integrated with national information databases (such as prescription drug information systems) and local hospital and primary-care systems.

Although these envisioned innovations hold great promise, they will render current V&V processes obsolete. Unless new certification technologies are developed and unless V&V processes undergo a paradigm shift, innovation will be stifled, because manufacturers and regulators will find the V&V of systems too costly—or we will see dramatic increases in security breaches and harmful incidents due to device malfunction.

What Can We Do Well?

Designing bug-free software is difficult—especially in complex devices that may be used in unanticipated contexts. Existing practices have worked as well as they have because industry V&V personnel and regulators take their jobs seriously.

We know how to develop and regulate **standalone and embedded medical devices** that have moderate complexity and are based on mature technology. In such cases, the domain is generally well understood, and the technology provides a level of confidence because the evolution of devices is incremental.

Wallace and Kuhn, in "Lessons from 342 Medical Device Failures," clearly indicate that many failures could be prevented just by systematically employing known quality assurance techniques.

Industry seems to perform the following V&V activities reasonably well:

- Gathering requirements
- Coding
- Testing
- Performing hazard analysis

In particular, collective knowledge and experience within large, well-established companies aid the effort necessary to prepare for validation activities.

The adoption of state-of-the-art techniques for software development is not uniform across the industry. Some companies are beginning to incorporate advanced design techniques into their development processes. Guidant, for example, uses rich modeling tools and product-line architectures to develop its pacemaker software. Clean-room software engineering and modeling have also had some success.

Automated tools for V&V activities—ranging from homegrown configuration management systems to static analysis tools—can have wide-ranging benefits. They can raise overall quality by reducing the risk of human error in applying quality assurance techniques and by reducing the time and effort needed to apply the techniques. A reduction of time and effort can free up resources that can be applied to obtain greater and denser coverage of code and to encourage innovation and technological advances by speeding up time to market.

Why Can't We Declare Victory?

Despite the pluses listed in the previous section, existing technology faces many challenges:

> **Lack of Tools that Automate Certification Tasks.** Generally, we know how to perform activities such as writing requirements, prototyping, and testing, but we need to perform them more accurately and in a more automated way. We also need to achieve greater cross- leveraging of techniques and artifacts—that is, we need to create architectures and processes that allow the information produced by one tool to

supplement and increase the effectiveness of other tools. Currently, almost all tools are standalone tools and are not context aware.

Large-Scale, Complex Devices Stress Current Best Practices. We are still challenged by large-scale, complex devices, such as proton therapy facilities. For these types of devices, the validation procedures and test cases can number in the hundreds of thousands. The burden of validation—in time and costs—slows the time to bring devices to market. Engineers often feel overwhelmed by complexity.

Limited and Ad Hoc Systems Integration. We are able to integrate products developed by a single manufacturer. But in a clinical environment, people are incorporating devices from different manufacturers, and technical personnel must be trained to recognize potential incompatibilities.

Inability to Capture and Model Clinical Environments and Processes. The correct operation of many devices relies on assumptions about the clinical environment or process in which the devices will be used. We are experiencing device failures due to unexpected interferences between devices and environments. Clear specifications of environmental assumptions and processes are needed. Formal models are preferred because they would enable tool integration.

Lack of Component-Based Approaches to Certification. Current V&V procedures focus on approving complete devices or systems—not components of systems. The emphasis is on end-to-end testing against device requirements. No regulatory mechanism allows reusable, individually deployable components or infrastructure to be certified in a way that reduces overall certification costs when the components are used in larger systems.

Inadequate Coverage of Security Issues in Certification. In today's V&V of devices, security issues are almost never considered. Yet the increasing blending of devices, medical records, telemedicine, and home, local, regional, and national networks will make security a central concern in the certification of future systems.

Widely Varying Knowledge and Training Across Vendors. Although some device vendors use state-of-the-art development practices and quality assurance techniques, many are uninformed about best practices for techniques such as test case generation, testing to different coverage metrics, and capturing requirements. Indeed, studies have concluded that the nature of many reported device faults indicates that known practices may have been misused or may not have been used at all. Moreover, clinical engineers receive little formal training—they gain knowledge through experience.

Device Interference and Poor Integration. Industry is doing fairly well at integrating products developed by a single manufacturer (such as Varian's Linac, used in concert with imaging devices and treatment planning systems). As the benefits of system integration are realized, however, and as integration mechanisms become commonplace in other domains, such as the highly successful and widely used universal serial bus (USB) from the personal- computer domain, the number of attempts to connect and integrate devices is increasing significantly. Such integrations are largely proceeding ad hoc, with little or no documentation and no systematic training.

Specific R&D Challenges

Based on the assessment presented above, we now lay out specific R&D challenges associated with certification.

Formulating Requirements

The development process begins by formulating requirements. The requirements formulation phase is the most important and one of the most-challenging-to-execute phases of development for medical devices.

We need technologies that support more automated and rigorous methods of eliciting and capturing requirements as described by experts in their respective domains. We also need technologies that can leverage requirements, including technologies that—

Directly perform semantic querying or simulation of use cases
Derive test cases more effectively and automatically from requirements
Generate visualizations and natural-language descriptions from requirements
Generate artifacts and reports needed for certification directly from requirements

Not only must we capture requirements that are appropriate; we must also automate capabilities for assessing and evaluating requirements.

Modeling and Formalizing Clinical Environments and Processes

One trend in the practice of medicine is a proliferation of sophisticated devices in complex environments where exceptions are the norm. We must develop a more rigorous approach to capturing, visualizing, and reasoning about clinical environments and processes. In particular, research should address the following questions:

How do we incorporate variability in clinical environments?
Can we mine rigorous descriptions of processes, workflows, and so forth to guide the development of device requirements or detect problematic device interaction in a clinical environment?
Can we use those models to clarify goals and focus the tasks to achieve more rigorous clinical validation?

Benefiting from Automated Tool Support

The FDA has relied on device manufacturers to validate the tools they use to develop their devices. Generally, manufacturers accomplish this by validating that a finished device performs as intended and by making sure that tool patches are up to date. But the scope of the validation process is limited. As devices become more complex and interconnected, more attention will need to be paid to tools' comprehensiveness and trustworthiness. We have opportunities to borrow from other industry sectors. For example, the FDA might recognize tools from the aviation domain that have been DO-178B certified or that conform to European MISRA coding and compiler standards.

Moreover, the lack of integration or synergistic interplay between tools and the encompassing development process means that some potential benefits of automated tool support are unrealized. Tools could be enhanced with standardized reporting formats that the FDA recognizes and that could support automated querying and auditing by FDA regulators—greatly increasing regulators' efficiency and accuracy.

Reorienting Procedures Toward Component-Based Certification

The development of component-based software—software that has individually deployable and reusable components—can reduce software development costs. Some vendors are effectively developing large-scale software systems by using *product-line* methods, in which the cost of developing *families* of similar systems is reduced by identifying commonalities across all systems in a family and then developing common components. Current development trends, along with the need to support emerging plug-and-play devices, provide a clear mandate to develop component-based approaches to certification.

Developing Safety-Critical Middleware

Closely tied to component-based certification and the use of product lines is the need for high- assurance and safety-critical middleware. Middleware is system software that resides between applications and the underlying operating systems, network protocol stacks, and hardware. It is often described as the "glue code" or "plumbing" that hooks multiple applications together and routes data and information transparently between different back-end sources of data.

The development of sophisticated plug-and-play devices, devices integrated through networks, and systems of systems as in operating rooms of the future will all require reusable infrastructure code that deals with the complexities of distributed systems. Middleware technology such as Common Object Request Broker Architecture (CORBA) provides a development solution.

Unfortunately, most middleware implementations use complex object-oriented design patterns that are difficult to validate. We need safety-critical middleware implementations, which vendors are reluctant to pursue because of an uncertain market. Changes in regulatory guidelines might encourage the production of safety-critical middleware.

Certifying in the Presence of Change

Obtaining certification for upgrades or changes to already "certified" products is costly and error prone. Many failures occur because of the inadequate recertification of modified devices. The state of the art for medical device recertification does not include the use of tools from programming language and software engineering—such as program slicers, dependence analysis, and impact analysis—that could be applied to determine exactly which sections of a software implementation are affected by modifications to code and to requirements.

Researchers should pursue more sophisticated techniques for dependence analysis, which could help determine the impact of changes. Potential examples are techniques that manage certification artifacts and automatically detect where rework in the presence of change is necessary. FDA recognition of tools that perform impact analysis and traceability could reduce the effort needed for retesting and recertification.

Monitoring Deployed Devices

We are able to report and track device "incidents," but reporting, tracking, publicizing, and interpreting the root causes of device incidents across manufacturers is problematic. We need to incorporate some notion of a "flight recorder" black-box reporting mechanism to gather data about events. Some devices, such as the Varian Linac, already incorporate "flight recorder" technology. Research is needed into runtime monitoring approaches that can be used in real-time embedded systems to gather event and fault data from medical devices. Statistical and sampling- based approaches to mining data collected from devices are also important.

Moving from Process-Driven Approval to Evidence-Based Certification

FDA device approval centers on a *process-driven* approach, in which manufacturers obtain approval by showing that they have carried out established quality assurance techniques such as code coverage, manual code inspections, and test cases. The approach often fails to account for innovations in development and verification techniques and does not encourage them. Moreover, as systems become more complex, we expect that best-effort processes will increasingly fail to catch subtle errors.

Research is needed into the alternate paradigm of an *evidence-based* approach, championed by John Rushby in his HCMDSS position paper, "Goal-Based Certification for Medical Devices." Instead of seeking to provide evidence that a process has been planned for and followed, the evidence-based approach seeks to generate independently verifiable evidence that a system satisfies its requirements. An example of a certification process based on an evidence-based or goal-based approach is the UK Defense Standard 00-56.

Formalizing Environment Models and Assumptions about Context

Device manufacturers often work under the assumption that devices will be used in certain fixed, step-by-step processes and will have no interaction with other devices. But when devices are used in environments that differ from those envisioned by the manufacturers, the devices often behave in unanticipated ways. An example is patients who have characteristics that deviate significantly from the norm (such as severely obese patients).

The state of the art relies on resolving undocumented and unanticipated interactions on the fly and in an ad hoc manner. Specifically, constraints on interactions are not captured in the validation process. As the number of devices in a clinical environment increases, and as the sophistication of devices and their connectivity methods (such as wireless Internet and Bluetooth radio) increases, clinical technicians will become overwhelmed with the task of assembling a safe and effective environment. Formalized models are needed of clinic environments, clinical processes, and assumptions made about the contexts in which devices will be deployed.

Dealing Effectively with the Certification of Security

Security-related research is needed in the following areas:

- Specification formalisms for specifying security properties at the level of system requirements, designs, and implementations
- Tools and techniques, such as those based on static analysis and lightweight theorem-proving, that can help verify that implementations satisfy specifications for security
- Regulatory guidelines, architecture recommendations, and techniques for security certification (Common Criteria and software architectures, for instance), to achieve standards such as the Multiple Independent Levels of Security (MILS) architecture

Research Strategies and Roadmap

It is likely that individual research teams can make progress in addressing the R&D challenges described above. Yet overall research progress and an exchange of ideas about research approaches, domain knowledge, and the effectiveness of competing techniques will be significantly hampered unless we can create significant infrastructure to support research on high-confidence medical devices.

Specifically, we need an infrastructure that facilitates interaction between device vendors and academic researchers. Researchers will be better able to address certification challenges facing V&V technologies if they have a detailed understanding of the certification process. Currently, researchers understand little about the certification process, and it makes little sense for them to engage in research about tools and techniques to aid certification or to propose changes in certification techniques without such an understanding.

These are two ideas to help researchers deepen their understanding of the certification process:

- FDA and industry hold training workshops on the review and approval process using example artifacts.
- FDA or industry performs a mock "red team" review process for products and artifacts developed by researchers. For example, the FDA or industry personnel could review medical device software built by academic researchers to demonstrate their V&V approaches. The review would use the same processes and standards that are applied to actual device submissions to the FDA.

The most important advances will come from the establishment of a research infrastructure, such as one or more open experimental platforms (OEP) for medical devices. An OEP is a publicly available test bed. In this instance, the OEP would provide realistic and complete examples of the following artifacts for a specific medical device:

- Requirements (including hazard analysis)
- Implementation or partial implementation
- Results of fault analysis, test cases, and other V&V activities
- Examples of material that would be submitted to the FDA for device approval

The OEP should also include a list of challenge problems, written by FDA and industry for academic researchers, that target areas on which researchers should focus. Strong consideration should be given to having national funding agencies contract with device vendors to—

- Develop OEP artifacts and challenge problems as described above
- Field questions from academic researchers
- Help evaluate tools and techniques that academic researchers have produced for realistic products and in realistic development settings

Five-Year Roadmap

The five-year roadmap involves the further development and maturation of tools that can provide automation for V&V and certification activities, including an initial exploration of V&V, the development of V&V techniques, and a demonstration of their usefulness. It would include the following steps:

- Develop an OEP for medical devices
- Apply existing process modeling languages to model clinical environments and processes
- Develop suites of sophisticated requirements for capturing, simulating, and querying requirements
- Incorporate more tools into the certification effort (adding value)
- Certify development tools (analysis and traceability tools) to reduce the burden of certification and recertification
- Enhance conventional formal method tools (static analysis and model-checking) to produce a variety of artifacts, including test cases and natural-language description of traceability steps
- Demonstrate the pervasive use of model-based development techniques with automated reasoning for—
  1. Component conformance to interfaces
  2. Component capability based on checking interface capability
  3. End-to-end reasoning of system behavior
  4. Managing, integrating, and automatically generating certification artifacts

Ten-Year Roadmap

The ten-year roadmap focuses on refining tools for use by manufacturers and regulatory agencies, including component-based certification, reuse of certification assets, and reuse of "precertified" high-assurance middleware and other infrastructure:

- Reorient the certification process toward component-based certification
- Develop certified components as commodities
- Arrive at the pervasive use of secure, QoS-aware, fault-tolerant, certified middleware
- Achieve integrated, end-to-end, model-based development frameworks dealing with composition, evolution, and change

Effectively demonstrate the metrics and other items necessary to change industry and regulatory practices

Establish a wide body of interoperability standards

Build more sophisticated tools for compositional analysis

Design tools for compositional hazard analysis

Appendix 4. Acronyms Used in Workshop Participants' Report

AHRQ	Agency for Healthcare Research and Quality
API	application programming interface
CDRH	Center for Device and Radiological Health (FDA)
CIMIT	Center for the Integration of Medicine and Innovative Technology
CISC	complex instruction set computer
CORBA	Common Object Request Broker Architecture
COTS	commercial off-the-shelf
CPS	cyber-physical systems
CSIA	Cyber Security and Information Assurance
DARPA	Defense Advanced Research Projects Agency
DICOM/HL7	Digital Imaging and Communications in Medicine standard Health Level 7
DCS	Digital Control System
DO-178B	defines the guidelines for development of aviation software in the U.S.
EEC	European Economic Commission
HER	electronic health record
EKG	electrocardiogram
EMF	electromagnetic field
ER	emergency room (of a hospital)
European Directive 93 and 42 EC	- harmonized standard for medical devices
FDA	U.S. Food and Drug Administration
FPGA	field programmable gate array
GDP	gross domestic product
HCSS	High Confidence Software and Systems
HCMDCPS	High Confidence Medical Device Cyber-Physical Systems
HCMDSS	High Confidence Medical Devices, Software, and Systems
HEC	High End Computing
HHS	U.S. Department of Health and Human Services
HIPAA	Health Insurance Portability and Accountability Act
HL7	Health Level 7, one of several American National Standards Institute (ANSI) -accredited Standards Developing Organizations that produces standards in the clinical and administrative healthcare arena
ICD	implantable cardiac defibrillator **ICU** - intensive care unit
IEC	International Electrotechnical Commission, an international standards and conformity assessment for government, business, and society for all electrical, electronic and related technologies

IEC 60601	a family of standards that specify requirements for electrical medical devices
IEEE	Institute of Electrical and Electronics Engineers
IEEE 1073/ISO 11073	an IEEE/ISO standard that defines rules for connecting bedside devices so that they can exchange data
ISO	International Standards Organization
ISO 9001	a standard for a general quality- management system
ISO 13407	a standard for a user-centered design process
ISO 13485	an ISO standard for quality- management systems that defines rules for assessing the robustness of a medical-device developer's quality-assurance processes
ISO 14971	an ISO standard that defines the components of a medical-device risk- management process
IT	information technology
ITK	Insight Toolkit, an open-source software toolkit for performing registration and segmentation
J2EE	Java 2 Platform Edition - defines the standard for developing multitier enterprise applications
LSN	Large Scale Networking
MDA	model-driven architecture
MDD	Medical Device Directive (e.g., MDD 93/42/EEC)
MD PnP	Medical Device Plug-and-Play
MEMS	micro-electromechanical systems
MILS	Multiple Independent Levels of Security
MISRA	EU-based Motor Industry Software reliability Association
NCO/NITRD	National Coordination Office for Networking and Information Technology Research and Development
NEMS	nano-electromechanical systems
NIH	National Institutes of Health
NIST	National Institute of Standards and Technology
NITRD	Networking and Information Technology Research and Development
NSA	National Security Agency
NSTC	National Science and Technology Council
NSF	National Science Foundation
ONCHI	Office of the National Coordinator for Health Information Technology
OEP	open experimental platform
OR	operating room
PACS	picture archive and communication systems
PC	personal computer
PCA	Program Component Area
PnP	plug and play
QoS	quality of service
QSR	Quality System Regulation (21 CFR 820, Oct. 7, 1996) - based on the ISO 9001 and ISO 13485 quality-system standards

R&D	research and development
RIM	Reference Information Model
RISC	reduced instruction set computer
SCADA	supervisory control and data acquisition
SEW	Social, Economic, and Workforce Implications of IT and IT Workforce Development
SOC	system on a chip
SOUP	software of unknown pedigree
TATRC	U.S. Army Telemedicine & Advanced Technology Research Center
TinyOS	An open-source operating system designed for wireless embedded sensor networks
UML	Unified Modeling Language
USB	universal serial bus
UWB	ultra-wideband
V&V	verification and validation
V&V&C	verification, validation, and certification

Appendix 5. Workshop Series Rosters

HCMDSS/MD PnP WORKSHOP 2007

Workshop Organizers
Julian M. Goldman, Massachusetts General
Hospital/Harvard Medical School (Co-Chair)
Insup Lee, University of Pennsylvania, (Co-Chair)
Oleg Sokolsky, University of Pennsylvania
Sue Whitehead, Center for the Integration of Medicine & Innovative Technology (CIMIT)

Sponsor Organizations and Points of Contact
AHRQ, J. Michael Fitzmaurice
NSF, Helen Gill and Sylvia Spengler
Partners Healthcare, Julian M. Goldman
TATRC, Ronald Marchessault
CIMIT, Julian Goldman and Sue Whitehead

Government Technical Advisors
Zohara Cohen, NIH David Du, NSF
Helen Gill, NSF
David Hislop, ARO
Paul Jones, FDA
Scott Midkiff, NSF
Sylvia Spengler, NSF
Sandy Weininger, FDA

Program Committee
Duncan Clarke, Fremont Associates
Rance Cleveland, University of Maryland Sherman Eagles, Medtronic, Inc.
Julian Goldman, Massachusetts General Hospital/Harvard Medical School
C. William Hanson, University of Pennsylvania School of Medicine
Jennifer Hou, University of Illinois at Urbana Champaign
S. Purushothaman Iyer, North Carolina State University
Jennifer Jackson, Brigham & Women's Hospital Biomedical Engineering
Insup Lee, University of Pennsylvania
Jane W.E. Liu, Academia Sinica, Taiwan ROC Steve Liu, Texas A&M University
George Pappas, University of Pennsylvania
James H. Philip, Harvard Medical School/Brigham and Women's Hospital
Victoria Rich, University of Pennsylvania School of Nursing
Majid Sarrafzadeh, UCLA
Rich Schrenker, Massachusetts Hospital Biomedical Engineering
Bren Seals, University of Kentucky Jack Stankovic, University of Virginia
Janos Sztipanovits, Vanderbilt University

Workshop Participants
Marwan Abdeen, McMaster University
Oscar Almeida, Texas A&M University
David Arney, University of Pennsylvania
Maxim Batalin, University of California, Los Angeles
Trudy E. Bell, NCO/NITRD
Jim Biondi, Cardiopulmonary Corporation Steven Boutus, CIMIT
Jeffrey Brown, Partners Health Care
Darin Buxbaum, Stanford University
Susan Carr, Patient Safety and Quality Healthcare
Orietam Celiku, Carnegie Mellon University
Yung-Chun Chen, University of Washington
Duncan Clarke, Fremont Associates, LLC Zohara Cohen, NIBIB/NIH
Philippe-Antoine Cortes, University of Pennsylvania
Steven Dain, University of Western
Ontario/University of Modena and Reggio Francesco De Mola, Emilia
Ann Demaree, CapsuleTech, Inc.
Robert Dingwell, The MITRE Corporation
Steve Dixon, Hill-Rom
Amy Droitcour, ALZA
Scott Eaton, Datascope Corporation
Ryam Eavey, Stryker
Jill Egeth, The MITRE Corporation
Javier Espina, Philips
Jim Fackler, Johns Hopkins University
Raimund Feldmann, Frauhnofer Center, Maryland
Jim Fidacaro, Datascope Corporation Gordon Fowler, DocBox, Inc.
Ken Fuchs, Draeger Medical Systems, Inc. John Garguilo, NIST

David Garlan, Carnegie Mellon University
Mark Gaynor, Boston University
Tim Gee, Medical Connectivity
Christopher Gilll, Washington University
Helen Gill, National Science Foundation
Gigi Gilman, Partners Healthcare
Julian M. Goldman, Massachusetts General Hospital
John Goodenough, Software Engineering Institute
Deniz Gurkan, University of Houston
Rick Hampton, Partners Healthcare System
Bryce Hayashida, Karl Storz Endoscopy
America, Inc.
John Hayes, University of Michigan
John Hedley-Whyte Harvard University
Dyke Hendrickson, CIMIT
Glenn Himes, MITRE Corporation
David Hislop, ARO (Retired)
Sally Howe, NCO/NITRD
Benedict Hui, University of Washington
May Lou Ingeholm, Georgetown University
Jennifer Jackson, Brigham & Women's Hospital
Roozbeh Jafari, University of Texas at Dallas
David Jea, UCLA
Raoul Jetley, FDA
Paul Jones, FDA
Tom Judd, Kaiser Permanente
Peter Kazanzides, Johns Hopkins University Arif Khan, Southcoast Hospitals Group
Ji Eun Kim, University of Pittsburgh Frankie Denise King, NCO/NITRD
Robert Kolodner, Department of Health & Human Services
Kai Kuck, Draegerwerk AG
Phillip Kuryloski, Cornell University
Ben Kwan, Polytechnic University
John LaCourse, University of New Hampshire
Patrick Lafleche, Stryker Medical
Brian Larson, Boston Scientific
Insup Lee, University of Pennsylvania Kathy Lesh, MITRE
Jane Liu, Academia Sinica
Steve Liu, Texas A&M University Donna Maddox, GE Healthcare
Manfred Maiers, ACIST Medical Systems Don Malackowski, Stryker
Rahul Mangharam, Carnegie Mellon University
Sowmya Manjanatha, Boston University Harry Manolopoulos, MiSim
Amen Ra Mashariki, Morgan State University Tammara Massey, UCLA
Martha Matzke, NCO/NITRD
Douglas Mcclure, Partners HealthCare
Robert McCready, The MITRE Corporation
Jay McGuire, Cardiopulmonary Corporation

Paul Mckneely, MediCAN Systems, Inc.
Yitzhak Mendelson, Worcester Polytechnic Nstitute
Joerg-Uwe Meyer, Draegerwerk AG
Scott Midkiff, NSF
Debra Milamed, Harvard Medical School
Austin Montgomery, Software Engineering Institute
In Mun, HCA
Ronald Newbower, CIMIT
Jeff Ojala, University of New Hampshire
Andrea O'Neill, ZOLL Medical
Jason Padvorac, University of Washington
John Parrish, CIMIT
Frederick Pearce, Walter Reed Army Institute of Research
Joshua Pearl, IXXAT, Inc.
Tomasz Petelenz, Sarcos Research Corp, University of Utah
Ken Peterson, Physio-Control, Inc.
James Phillip, Brigham & Women's Hospital
Raj Rajkumar, Carnegie Mellon, University
Steven Rakitin, Software Quality Consulting
Tracy Rausch, DocBox Inc.
Elaine Richardson, CIMIT
David Ristau, Northern Digital Inc.
Jeff Robbins, LiveData, Inc.
Michael Robkin, Kaiser Permanente
Kurt Rohloff, BBN Technologies
Harvey Rubin, University of Pennsylvania
John Rushby, SRI International
Vish Sankaran, HIT
Majid Sarrafzadeh, UCLA
Rick Schrenker, Massachusetts General Hospital
Jeff Scott, LiveData, Inc.
Brent Seales, University of Kentucky
Lui Sha, University of Illinois
Chi-Sheng Shih, National Taiwan University
Frank Sites, Hospital of the University of Pennsylvania
Harry Sleeper, The MITRE Corporation
Oleg Sokolsky, University of Pennsylvania
Juhan Sonin, The MITRE Corporation
Bill Spees, FDA
Sylvia Spengler, NSF
Soundararajan Srinivasan, Robert Bosch LLC
Mani Srivastava, UCLA
Binay Sugla, Mobile Matrix
Mu Sun, University of Illinois at Urbana- Champaign
Thomas Szabo, Boston University
Carl F. Wallroth, Draeger Medical, Inc. Jonathan Waters, University of New Hampshire

Sandy Weininger, US FDA
James Welch, Masimo
Susan Whitehead, CIMIT
Karl Wolf, McKesson Provider Technologies
Han-Chun Yeh, Academia Sinica
Raymond Zambuto, IHE-USA
Holger Zeltwanger, CAN in Automation

HCMDSS Workshop 2005

Workshop Organizers
Insup Lee (Co-Chair), University of Pennsylvania
George Pappas, University of Pennsylvania
Janos Sztipanovits, Vanderbilt University
Shankar, Sastry, University of California-Berkeley

Government Sponsor Agencies and Points of Contact
FDA, Paul Jones
NIST, Paul Black
NSA, William Bradley Martin
NSF, Helen Gill
NCO/NITRD, Sally Howe/Frankie King

Program Committee
Tarek Abdelzaher, University of Virginia
Rance Cleaveland, Reactive Systems, Inc.
Helen Gill, NSF
Julian M. Goldman, Massachusetts General Hospital/Harvard Medical School
John Hatcliff, Kansas State University Paul L. Jones, FDA
Bruce Krogh, Carnegie Mellon University
Insup Lee, University of Pennsylvania
Peter Lee, Carnegie Mellon University
Brian Litt, Hospital of University of Pennsylvania
Jane Liu, IIS, Academia Sinica, Taiwan
William Bradley Martin, NSA
George J. Pappas, University of Pennsylvania
Raj Rajkumar, Carnegie Mellon University
Victoria L. Rich, Hospital of University of Pennsylvania/School of Nursing
Douglas Rosendale, VA
Harvey Rubin, University of Pennsylvania School of Medicine
Doug Schmidt, Vanderbilt University
Janos Sztipanovits, Vanderbilt University

Workshop Participants

Tarek F. Abdelzaher, University of Virginia
Ashok Agrawala, University of Maryland
Rajeev Alur, University of Pennsylvania Madhukar Anand
David Arney
Ruzena Bajcsy, UC Berkeley
Douglas Barton, Lockheed Martin
Scott L. Bartow, Sentara Home Care Services
Poppy Rae Bass, University of Pennsylvania Hospital
Joseph Bergmann, The Open Group
M. Brian Blake, Georgetown University
Amit Bose, Tyco Healthcare – Puritan Bennett
Timothy Buchman, Washington University
Daniel N. Carozza, VA
Andrew Casertano, VA
M. Cenk Cavusoglu, Case Western Reserve University
W. Rance Cleaveland II, Reactive Systems Inc./University of Maryland
Peter Coronado, Varian Medical Systems
Rich Craft, Sandia National Laboratories
Kenneth C. Curley, TATRC
Ralph DePalma, VA Hospital
Steve Dimmer, Calypso Medical Technologies
Matthew Dwyer, University of Nebraska
Sherman Eagles, Medtronic, Inc.
Arvind Easwaran
Mike Eklund, UC Berkeley
Aaron Evans
George Fainekos
Sebastian Fischmeister
Jacob Flanz, Massachusetts General Hospital
Steven Getz, Animas Corporation
Chris Gill, Washington University
Helen Gill, NSF
Julian Goldman, Massachusetts General
Hospital/Harvard Medical School
Elsa L. Gunter, University of Illinois – Urbana Champaign
Sandeep K. S. Gupta, Arizona State University
John Hatcliff, Kansas State University
Scott Henninger, University of Nebraska at Lincoln
David W. Hislop, Army Research Office
Jennifer C. Hou, University of Illinois – Urbana Champaign
Zachary Ives, University of Pennsylvania
David R. Jones, Philips Medical Systems
LeRoy Jones, HHS/ONCHIT
Mark P. Jones, Oregon Heath & Science University
Paul L. Jones, FDA

Nagarajan Kandasamy, Drexel University
Soon Ju Kang , Kyungpook National University
Frankie Denise King, NCO/NITRD T. John Koo, Vanderbilt University
Robert C. Kircher, Dose Safety Company
Bruce H. Krogh, Carnegie Mellon University
Peter M. Kuzmak, VA
Insup Lee, University of Pennsylvania
Peter Lee, Carnegie Mellon University
Jane W. S. Liu, IIS, Academia Sinica, Taiwan
Ronald Marchessault, TATRC
Brad Martin, NSA
Tom Martin, Virginia Tech
Rami Melhem, University of Pittsburgh
Douglas Miller, Massachusetts General Hospital
Klara Nahrstedt, University of Illinois at Urbana-Champaign
Jens Palsberg, UCLA
George Pappas, University of Pennsylvania
Tomasz Petelenz, Sarcos Research Corporation
Rosemary C. Polomano
Stacy Prowell, University of Tennessee
Raj Rajkumar, Carnegie Mellon University
John Regehr, University of Utah
Victoria Rich, University of Pennsylvania Hospital
Michael Robkin, Kaiser Permanente
Douglas Rosendale, VA
Gregg Rothermel, University of Nebraska
Harvey Rubin, University of Pennsylvania
John Rushby, SRI, International
Vish Sankaran, HHS/ONCHIT
Tariq Samad, Honeywell Labs
Majid Sarrafzadeh, UCLA
Rich Schrenker, Massachusetts General Hospital
Lui Sha, University of Illinois – Urbana Champaign
Gregory Sharp, Massachusetts General Hospital
Oleg Sokolsky, University of Pennsylvania
Sang Son, University of Virginia
Jack Stankovic, University of Virginia
Simon Szykman, NCO/NITRD
Charles A. Taylor, Stanford University
Russell Taylor, Johns Hopkins University
Steve Van Albert, Walter Reed Army Instituteof Research
Bow-Yaw Wang, IIS, Academia Sinica
Wei Zhao, ((Rensalier Polytechnic Institute (NSF at the time of the workshop))
Taieb Znati, NSF (University of Pittsburgh at the time of the workshop)

NCO/NITRD Coordination Contributors
Vivian Harris
Sally Howe
Frankie King

HCMDSS Planning Workshop 2004

Workshop Organizers
Insup Lee, University of Pennsylvania
George Pappas, University of Pennsylvania
Janos Sztipanovits, Vanderbilt University

Government Sponsor Agencies and Points of Contact
NCO/NITRD, Sally Howe/Frankie King

Program Committee
Helen Gill, NSF
Sally Howe, NCO/NITRD
Frankie King, NCO/NITRD
Shankar Sastry, UC Berkeley
Janos Sztipanovits, Vanderbilt University
Insup Lee, University of Pennsylvania
George Pappas, University of Pennsylvania

Workshop Participants
Felix Alfonso, Defense Blood Standard System
Lutz Andersohn, Nellcor/Tyco Healthcare
John Anton, Kestrel Institute
Anindya Banerjee, Kansas State University
Scott Bartow, Sentara Home Care Services
Nekeia Bell, NCO/NITRD
Joseph Bergmann, The Open Group
Paul Black, National Institute of Standards and Technology (NIST)
Mike Blomquist, Smiths Medical Medication Delivery & Patient Monitoring
Amit Bose, Nellcor/Puritan Bennett
Andrew Casertano, Department of Veterans Affairs (VA)
Kevin Cleary, Imaging Science and
Information Systems (ISIS) Center
Rance Cleaveland, Reactive Systems, Inc.
Peter Coronado, Varian Medical Systems
Vincent Crum, AFRL/VACC
Ralph De Palma, Veterans Administration Hospital
David Forslund, Cognition Group
Robert Galloway, Vanderbilt University
Ronald Gerner, Abbott Laboratories

Helen Gill, National Science Foundation
Julian M. Goldman, Massachusetts General Hospital / Harvard Medical School
Karl Hammermeister, University of Colorado Health Sciences Center
John Hatcliff, Kansas State University
Ron Hensel, Department of Veterans Affairs
David Hislop, U.S. Army Research Office
Sally Howe, NCO/NITRD
Edmond Israelski, Abbott Laboratories
Purush Iyer, NC State University
Mark Jones, Oregon Health & Science University (OGI)
Paul Jones, U.S. Food and Drug Administration
Peter Kazanzides, Johns Hopkins University
Frankie Denise King, NCO/NITRD
Robert Kircher, Dose Safety Company
Lori Lazzara, Philips Medical Systems
Insup Lee, University of Pennsylvania
Peter Lee, Carnegie Mellon University
Eric Linner, Baxter Healthcare
Brian Litt, University of Pennsylvania
Jane Liu, IIS, Academia Sinica, Taiwan
Daniel Maloney, Veterans Hospital
Administration (VHA)
Martha Matzke, NCO/NITRD
Virginia Moore, NCO/NITRD
George Pappas, University of Pennsylvania
Michael Parsons, Computerized Medical Systems
Tomasz Petelenz, Sarcos Research Corporation
Jesse Poore, University of Tennessee
Stacy Prowell, University of Tennessee
Raj Rajkumar, Carnegie Mellon University
Sohan Ranjan, Georgetown University
Victoria Rich, Hospital of the University of Pennsylvania
Douglas Rosendale, Veterans Affairs Office of Information and Surgery
Harvey Rubin, University of Pennsylvania
Doug Schmidt, Vanderbilt University
Russell Taylor, Johns Hopkins University
Alan Tellington, NCO/NITRD
Majed Tomeh, QCMetrix, Inc.
Vy Tran, Varian Medical Systems
Steve Van Albert, Walter Reed Army Institute of Research
Nicholas Wright, NCO/NITRD
John Zaleski, Siemens Medical Solutions Health Services

NCO/NITRD Coordination Contributors
Nekeia Bell
Sally Howe

Frankie King
Virginia Moore
Allen Tellington

Appendix 6. Acknowledgments

The authors of this Government report extend sincerest appreciation to the many academic and industry experts in the high-confidence IT R&D community who planned and participated in the medical-device workshop series and developed the 2006 workshop participants' report. Through their intensive intellectual engagement over time, these contributors articulated and shaped the theoretical, scientific, and technical framework for the research agenda discussed in our report.

We look forward to continuing this fruitful nationwide collaboration toward truly high-confidence cyber-physical systems for 21st century health care.

We also thank the NCO/NITRD staff, which played an instrumental role in the development of our report, including assisting in research, editing and rewriting text, and publishing the final document.

Cover design

James L. Caras, Scientific Designer/Illustrator, Design and Publishing Division, National Science Foundation

Image credits

Front cover – Photo by Steve Wood, courtesy of the University of Alabama-Birmingham

Back cover (from left to right/top to bottom) – Photos courtesy of:

University of Florida Neuroprosthetics Research Group; U.S. Air Force; Sandia National Laboratory; Siemens press pictures; U.S. Veterans Administration; Southern Health Diagnostic Imaging, Australia; Beaumont Hospitals, Royal Oak, Mich.; the University of Washington (images of prosthetic hand and researcher Yoky Matsuoka with prosthetic finger); U.S. Army; and U.S. Centers for Disease Control.

End Notes

[1] This report uses the term "high confidence" to encompass the behavior of hardware, software, and systems (devices) regardless of size or complexity, plus all interconnections; high-confidence systems are robust (manage failures) and can justifiably be trusted, especially when used in life-, safety-, security, and mission-critical situations. Note that this definition applies to individual components and their interconnections, to software, hardware, and systems at all levels, and potentially also to a nationwide infrastructure.

[2] AHRQ and TATRC were Federal co-sponsors of the June 2007 workshop.

[3] The U.S. medical devices sector includes surgical and medical instruments, orthopedic, prosthetic, and surgical appliances and supplies; dental equipment and supplies; x-ray apparatus, tubes, related irradiation apparatus; electrotherapy and electromedical apparatus; ophthalmic equipment; and in-vitro diagnostic substances. Annual Survey of Manufacturers, 2006, U.S. Census Bureau, Department of Commerce.

[4] Annual Survey of Manufacturers, 2006, U.S. Census Bureau, Department of Commerce.

[5] See discussion in *Software for Dependable Systems: Sufficient Evidence?*, National Academies Press, Washington, D.C., 2007

[6] Annual Survey of Manufacturers, 2006, U.S. Census Bureau, Department of Commerce.

[7] Medical Device Industry Assessment, 2008, International Trade Commission, Department of Commerce.

[8] The growing elderly population in the United States is viewed as a key influence on the direction of the medical device industry. A Profile of Older Americans: 2007, Administration on Aging, U.S. Department of Health and Human Services.

[9] "Open-loop" is used throughout this report to refer to systems that lack feedback control; "closed-loop" refers to systems that include feedback control.

[10] The phrase "open systems" is used to describe systems designed to allow ready interconnection and interoperation with other systems; "closed systems" refers to those designed to be used in isolation.

[11] National Academies Press, *op. cit.*

[12] *Leadership Under Challenge: Information Technology R&D in a Competitive World*, President's Council of Advisors on Science and Technology, August 2007, p. 31.

[13] Annual Survey of Manufacturers, 2006, U.S. Census Bureau, Department of Commerce.

Chapter 2

FDA Should Take Steps to Ensure that High-Risk Device Types are Approved through the Most Stringent Premarket Review Process*

United Stated Government Accountability Office

Why GAO Did This Study

The Food and Drug Administration (FDA) within the Department of Health and Human Services (HHS) is responsible for oversight of medical devices sold in the United States. Regulations place devices into three classes, with class III including those with the greatest risk to patients. Unless exempt by regulation, new devices must clear FDA premarket review via either the 510(k) premarket notification process, which determines if a new device is substantially equivalent to another legally marketed device, or the more stringent premarket approval (PMA) process, which requires the manufacturer to supply evidence providing reasonable assurance that the device is safe and effective. Class III devices must generally obtain an approved PMA, but until FDA issues regulations requiring submission of PMAs, certain types of class III devices may be cleared via the 510(k) process. The FDA Amendments Act of 2007 mandated that GAO study the 510(k) process. GAO examined which premarket review process—510(k) or PMA—FDA used to review selected types of device submissions in fiscal years 2003 through 2007. GAO reviewed FDA data and regulations, and interviewed FDA officials.

---

* This is an edited, reformatted and augmented version of a U. S. Government Accountability Office publication dated January 2009.

What GAO Recommends

GAO recommends that FDA expeditiously take steps to issue regulations for class III device types currently allowed to enter the market via the 510(k) process by requiring PMAs or reclassifying them to a lower class. HHS agreed with GAO's recommendation.

What GAO Found

In fiscal years 2003 through 2007, as part of its premarket review to determine whether devices should be permitted to be marketed in the United States, FDA

reviewed 13,199 submissions for class I and II devices via the 510(k) process, clearing 11,935 (90 percent) of these submissions;
reviewed 342 submissions for class III devices through the 510(k) process, clearing 228 (67 percent) of these submissions; and
reviewed 217 original and 784 supplemental PMA submissions for class III devices and approved 78 percent and 85 percent, respectively, of these submissions.

Although Congress envisioned that class III devices would be approved through the more stringent PMA process, and the Safe Medical Devices Act of 1990 required that FDA either reclassify or establish a schedule for requiring PMAs for class III device types, this process remains incomplete. GAO found that in fiscal years 2003 through 2007 FDA cleared submissions for 24 types of class III devices through the 510(k) process. As of October 2008, 4 of these device types had been reclassified to class II, but 20 device types could still be cleared through the 510(k) process. FDA officials said that the agency is committed to issuing regulations either reclassifying or requiring PMAs for the class III devices currently allowed to receive clearance for marketing via the 510(k) process, but did not provide a time frame for doing so.

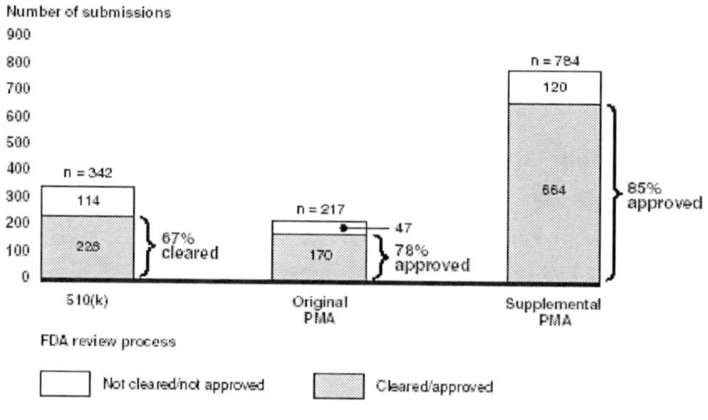

Source: GAO analysis of FDA data.

Notes: *510(k)* includes traditional and abbreviated 510(k) submissions. *Supplemental PMA* includes certain types of submissions for changes to devices that were previously approved through the PMA process. *Not cleared/not approved* includes 510(k) submissions that were denied or other (e.g., withdrawn) and PMAs that were withdrawn or otherwise not approved.

Class III Device Submissions with FDA Review Decisions in Fiscal Years 2003 through 2007, by FDA Review Process and Review Decision

Abbreviations

FDA	Food and Drug Administration
FDCA	Federal Food, Drug, and Cosmetic Act
HHS	Department of Health and Human Services
NSE	not substantially equivalent
PMA	premarket approval
SE	substantially equivalent
SMDA	Safe Medical Devices Act of 1990

January 15, 2009

The Honorable Edward M. Kennedy
Chairman
The Honorable Michael B. Enzi
Ranking Member
Committee on Health, Education, Labor, and Pensions
United States Senate

The Honorable Henry A. Waxman
Chairman
The Honorable Joe Barton
Ranking Member
Committee on Energy and Commerce
House of Representatives

The Honorable Charles E. Grassley
United States Senate

The Honorable John D. Dingell
House of Representatives

The federal government, through the Food and Drug Administration (FDA) within the Department of Health and Human Services (HHS), is responsible for ensuring that medical devices sold in the United States provide reasonable assurance of safety and effectiveness and do not pose a threat to public health.[1] These devices range from simple tools like bandages and surgical clamps to complicated devices like pacemakers.

FDA classifies each device type into one of three classes—class I, II, or III—based on the level of risk it poses and the controls necessary to reasonably ensure its safety and effectiveness.[2] According to FDA, the risk the type of device poses to the patient or the user is a major factor in the class it is assigned: class I includes devices with the lowest risk, and class III includes devices with the highest risk. Examples of types of devices in each class include the following:

class I: tongue depressors, elastic bandages, reading glasses, and forceps;
class II: electrocardiographs, powered bone drills, and mercury thermometers; and
class III: pacemakers and replacement heart valves.

In general, unless exempt under FDA regulations, devices are subject to one of two types of FDA premarket review before they may be legally marketed in the United States.[3]

Premarket approval (PMA): The manufacturer must provide evidence, typically including clinical data, providing reasonable assurance that the new device is safe and effective. The PMA process is the most stringent type of premarket review. A successful submission results in FDA approval.

Premarket notification (510(k)): The manufacturer must demonstrate to FDA that the new device is *substantially equivalent* to a device already legally on the market that does not require a PMA.[4] A successful submission results in FDA clearance.[5]

In general, class I and II device types subject to premarket review are required to obtain FDA clearance through the 510(k) process, and class III device types are required to obtain FDA approval through the more stringent PMA process. However, certain types of class III devices that were in commercial distribution in the United States before May 28, 1976[6] (called preamendment device types) and those determined to be substantially equivalent to them may be cleared through the less stringent 510(k) process until FDA publishes regulations requiring them to go through the PMA process or reclassifies them into a lower class.[7] The Safe Medical Devices Act of 1990 (SMDA) required FDA (1) to reexamine the preamendment class III device types for which PMAs were not yet required to determine if they should be reclassified to class I or II or remain in class III and (2) to establish a schedule to promulgate regulations requiring those preamendment device types that remain in class III to obtain FDA approval through the PMA process.[8] Accordingly, all class III devices are eventually to be reviewed through the PMA process.

The FDA Amendments Act of 2007[9] mandated that GAO study FDA's premarket review of devices under section 510(k) of the Federal Food, Drug, and Cosmetic Act (FDCA).[10] This report discusses (1) the premarket review process—510(k) or PMA—FDA used to review class I, II, and III device submissions in fiscal years 2003 through 2007 and (2) the extent to which FDA has determined that devices reviewed through the 510(k) process had new intended uses or new technological characteristics.

To determine the premarket review process FDA used to review class I, II, and III device submissions, as well as the number of submissions reviewed and cleared in fiscal years 2003 through 2007, we obtained and analyzed data from FDA's 510(k) and PMA databases. These databases contain information on 510(k) and PMA submissions,[11] respectively, including the name of the device, the FDA-assigned product code,[12] the status of the submission, and any FDA decisions related to the submission and the dates of those decisions. We also used data from FDA's Device Nomenclature Management System to determine other attributes of the device types covered by the 510(k) and PMA submissions. We obtained and analyzed data on submissions for which FDA made review decisions in fiscal years 2003 through 2007.[13] Our analysis included traditional and abbreviated 510(k) submissions, original PMA submissions, and submissions for certain types of PMA supplements (panel-track and 180-day user-fee supplements).[14] To assess the reliability of these data, we interviewed FDA officials knowledgeable about these databases, performed electronic testing for accuracy and completeness, and where applicable compared our results to aggregate information from other sources, such as published FDA reports and the FDA Web site. We determined that the data were sufficiently reliable for the purposes of this report.[15]

To examine the extent to which FDA has determined that devices reviewed through the 510(k) process had new intended uses or new technological characteristics, we used FDA's 510(k) database to select and review all class III 510(k) submission files and a stratified random sample of class II 510(k) submission files for which FDA reached a determination of substantially equivalent (SE) or not substantially equivalent (NSE) in fiscal years 2005 through 2007. The sample totaled 459 submissions to the Office of Device Evaluation within FDA's Center for Devices and Radiological Health and did not include submissions to other FDA offices or centers.[16] In each case, we collected data primarily from the FDA reviewer's memo, which outlined the decisions that FDA made to reach its determination and summarized FDA's rationale for finding the submission SE or NSE. Because our sample of class II device submissions is representative of all class II device submissions meeting our selection criteria, in reporting the results of our analysis we provide estimates for the universe of all 4,900 traditional and abbreviated 510(k) submissions for class II devices for which FDA made determinations of SE or NSE in fiscal years 2005 through 2007. To assess the reliability of the data we obtained from FDA's files, we compared our results with information from FDA's 510(k) database. In addition, we discussed cases where the determination path or rationale was unclear with knowledgeable FDA officials. We determined that the data were sufficiently reliable for the purposes of this report.

In addition to our data analysis, we reviewed relevant laws, regulations, and FDA guidance, and interviewed FDA officials, representatives of professional associations representing device manufacturers, and consumer advocates. We conducted this performance audit from March 2008 to January 2009 in accordance with generally accepted government auditing standards. Those standards require that we plan and perform the audit to obtain sufficient, appropriate evidence to provide a reasonable basis for our findings and conclusions based on our audit objectives. We believe that the evidence obtained provides a reasonable basis for our findings and conclusions based on our audit objectives.

Results in Brief

In fiscal years 2003 through 2007, FDA reviewed all class I and II device submissions through the 510(k) process, and reviewed some types of class III device submissions through the 510(k) process and others through the PMA process.

FDA reviewed all 13,199 submissions for class I and class II devices through the 510(k) process, clearing 90 percent (11,935 submissions) for marketing.

FDA reviewed 342 submissions for class III devices through the 5 10(k) process, clearing 67 percent (228 submissions) for marketing.

> FDA also reviewed 217 original PMA submissions and 784 supplemental PMA submissions for class III devices, approving 78 percent and 85 percent, respectively, of these submissions for marketing.

Although Congress envisioned that class III devices would be approved through the more stringent PMA process, and the SMDA required that FDA establish a schedule for doing so, this process remains incomplete. We found that in the 5-year period we examined FDA cleared submissions for 24 class III device types through the 510(k) process. These submissions were more likely than class I or class II submissions to be implantable or life sustaining, or to pose a significant risk to the health, safety, or welfare of a patient. As of October 2008, 4 of the 24 device types had been reclassified and 20 class III device types could still be cleared through the 510(k) process. FDA officials have acknowledged the importance of publishing regulations requiring PMA submissions or reclassifying preamendment class III device types. When asked for their time frame for doing so, however, the officials did not provide one.

In fiscal years 2005 through 2007, FDA determined that relatively few class II and III devices reviewed through the 510(k) process had a new intended use or new technological characteristics. Of the 5,063 class II or class III 510(k) submissions with SE or NSE determinations in this time period, we estimate that about 1 percent had a new intended use and about 15 percent had new technological characteristics. Among devices FDA determined SE (and therefore cleared for marketing), all of the submissions had the same intended use and 86 percent had the same technological characteristics as a device already on the market. In contrast, among the 248 510(k) submissions found NSE, FDA determined that more than half of the devices had a new intended use or new technological characteristics.

We are recommending that FDA expeditiously take steps to issue regulations for each class III device type currently allowed to enter the market through the 510(k) process, including (1) reclassifying each device type into a lower class or requiring it to remain in class III and (2) for those device types remaining in class III, requiring approval for marketing through the PMA process. HHS commented that the draft report fairly and accurately describes the FDA's medical device 510(k) program and the department agreed with our conclusions and recommendation.

BACKGROUND

The Medical Device Amendments of 1976 established three classes of medical devices.[17] Under current law, these three device classes are defined as follows:

> Class I devices are those for which compliance with general controls, such as good manufacturing practices specified in FDA's quality system regulation, are sufficient to provide reasonable assurance of their safety and effectiveness.
>
> Class II devices are subject to general controls and may also be subject to special controls, such as postmarket surveillance, patient registries, or specific FDA guidelines, if general controls alone are insufficient to provide reasonable assurance of the device's safety and effectiveness.[18]

Class III devices are subject to general controls, but are distinguished from class I and II devices because class III devices are those (1) for which insufficient information exists to determine whether general and special controls are sufficient to provide a reasonable assurance of the safety and effectiveness of the device and (2) that support or sustain human life or are of substantial importance in preventing impairment of human health, or that present a potential unreasonable risk of illness or injury.

Devices Exempt from FDA Premarket Review

Under federal regulations, many types of devices are exempt from FDA premarket review.[19] Although FDA does not track the number of devices that are actually sold or marketed in the United States, manufacturers are required to register with FDA and provide a list of devices intended for commercial distribution, including device types that are exempt from premarket review.[20] As shown in figure 1, about 67 percent of the more than 50,000 separate devices that manufacturers listed with FDA during fiscal years 2003 through 2007 were exempt from premarket review.[21] Of the exempt devices that manufacturers listed with FDA, about 95 percent were class I devices, for example reading glasses and forceps. About 5 percent were class II devices, for example wheeled stretchers and mercury thermometers.

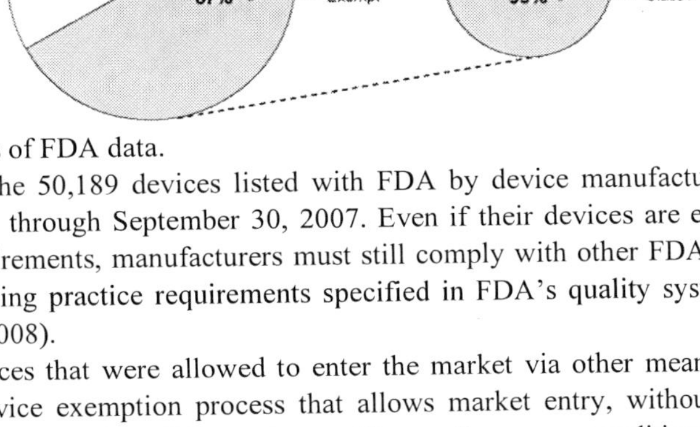

Source: GAO analysis of FDA data.

Notes: Data are for the 50,189 devices listed with FDA by device manufacturers during the period October 1, 2002, through September 30, 2007. Even if their devices are exempt from premarket notification requirements, manufacturers must still comply with other FDA requirements, such as good manufacturing practice requirements specified in FDA's quality system regulation. See 21 C.F.R. pt. 820 (2008).

[a] *Other* includes devices that were allowed to enter the market via other means, such as through the humanitarian device exemption process that allows market entry, without adherence to certain requirements, for devices benefiting patients with rare diseases or conditions.

Figure 1. Devices That Manufacturers Listed with FDA during Fiscal Years 2003 through 2007, by Review Process and Device Class

Premarket Review Process for Class III Devices

With the enactment of the Medical Device Amendments of 1976, Congress imposed requirements under which all class III devices would be approved through the PMA process before being marketed in the United States.[22] However, when it passed the 1976 amendments, Congress distinguished between those devices in commercial distribution before the date of enactment and those entering the market on or after enactment.

> **Preamendment devices.** Class III devices that were in commercial distribution prior to May 28, 1976 (referred to as preamendment devices) were allowed to be reviewed and cleared for the U.S. market without PMA approval until FDA published final regulations requiring each device type to obtain approval for the U.S. market through the PMA process.[23]
>
> **Postamendment devices.** Devices that were not in commercial distribution prior to May 28, 1976 (referred to as postamendment devices) were classified automatically into class III and required to go through the PMA process unless FDA either (1) determined they were substantially equivalent to a preamendment device type for which premarket approval is not required[24] or (2) reclassified the device type into class I or class II.[25]

Within this framework, Congress thus envisioned that class III devices would be approved through the more stringent PMA process and that the premarket review of class I and class II devices would entail a lesser degree of scrutiny.

By the late 1980s, FDA had not acted to require PMAs for many preamendment class III device types.[26] In 1990, the SMDA required FDA to

1. before December 1, 1995, order industry submission of safety and effectiveness information for preamendment class III device types that were not yet required to go through the PMA process;
2. after ordering industry submission of safety and effectiveness information but before December 1, 1995, publish regulations for each such device either revising its classification into class I or class II or requiring it to remain in class III;[27] and
3. as promptly as is reasonably achievable, but not later than 12 months after the effective date of a regulation requiring a device to remain in class III, establish a schedule for the promulgation of regulations requiring the submission of PMAs for the preamendment class III device types required to remain in class III.[28]

The House of Representatives report accompanying the SMDA stated that “In formulating these schedules, the FDA should take into account its priorities and limited resources, together with the Committee’s intention that the evaluation process be expeditious.”[29]

In May 1994, FDA published a notice in the *Federal Register* announcing a strategy for implementation of the SMDA.[30] According to the FDA memorandum outlining this strategy, the agency planned the following:

- To publish proposed regulations by 1996 requiring PMAs for 15 device types that FDA had determined to present an unreasonably high risk to public health because significant issues of safety or effectiveness or both were not being resolved or, to the best of FDA's knowledge, had little probability of being resolved. According to FDA, the timetable for publication of each final regulation would be based on specific data needs, comments received (in response to the proposed rule), and the existence, if any, of petitions received to reclassify the devices.
- To order manufacturers to submit information on safety and effectiveness by 1998 for 58 device types. FDA identified 27 of these device types as not presenting as great a risk to the public health in light of FDA's knowledge and experience with the devices. FDA identified the other 31 device types as strong candidates for reclassification. FDA's strategy stated that after receipt of the safety and effectiveness information, the agency would proceed with rule making to either reclassify the devices or retain them in class III.
- To issue one proposed regulation in 1994 requiring PMAs for 44 device types in limited use.

The agency's strategy established a plan to start addressing the class III device types that were allowed to go through the 510(k) process, but it did not establish completion dates for doing so. See appendix III for additional information on the FDA strategy.

FDA's 510(k) Review Process

As a general rule, devices are subject to 510(k) premarket review unless exempt or required to go through the PMA process. Specifically, the 5 10(k) process, established in 1976, requires a device manufacturer to notify FDA 90 days before it intends to market a device and to establish that the device is substantially equivalent to a legally marketed device that does not require a PMA. The legally marketed device is referred to as a predicate device. Under federal regulations, a predicate device can be a device that

- was legally marketed prior to May 28, 1976, for which a PMA is not required; or
- was marketed on or after May 28, 1976, and was found to be substantially equivalent to a legally marketed device through the 5 10(k) process; or
- was reclassified by FDA from class III to class II or I.[31]

FDA reviews each 510(k) submission to determine whether the device in question is SE or NSE to a predicate device.[32] To be SE, a device must (1) have the same intended use as the predicate device and (2) have the same technological characteristics as the predicate device or have different technological characteristics and submitted information demonstrates that the device is as safe and effective as the marketed device and does not raise different questions of safety or effectiveness. Because the predicate device may be a device that was marketed on or after May 28, 1976, that was found SE when compared to another legally marketed device through the 510(k) process, there could be multiple iterations of a given device type cleared through the 510(k) process. As a result, a 510(k) submission for a new device in 2008 could be compared to the 20th iteration of a device type that was on the market before 1976. Figure 2 shows FDA's 510(k) decision-making process.

Relative to the PMA process, the 510(k) premarket review process is generally:

> **Less stringent**. For most 510(k) submissions, clinical data are not required and substantial equivalence will normally be determined based on comparative device descriptions, including performance data.[33] In contrast, in order to meet the PMA approval requirement of providing reasonable assurance that a new device is safe and effective, most original PMAs and some PMA supplements require clinical data.[34] In addition, other aspects of FDA's premarket review are less stringent for 510(k) submissions than for PMA submissions. For example, FDA generally does not inspect manufacturing establishments as part of the 510(k) premarket review process—the 510(k) review process focuses primarily on the end product of the manufacturing process rather than the manufacturing process itself. In contrast, the agency does inspect manufacturing establishments as part of its review of original PMA submissions.[35] Manufacturing establishments that produce devices cleared through the 510(k) process, as well as those that produce devices approved through the PMA process, are subject to periodic inspections under FDA's normal inspection program.[36]

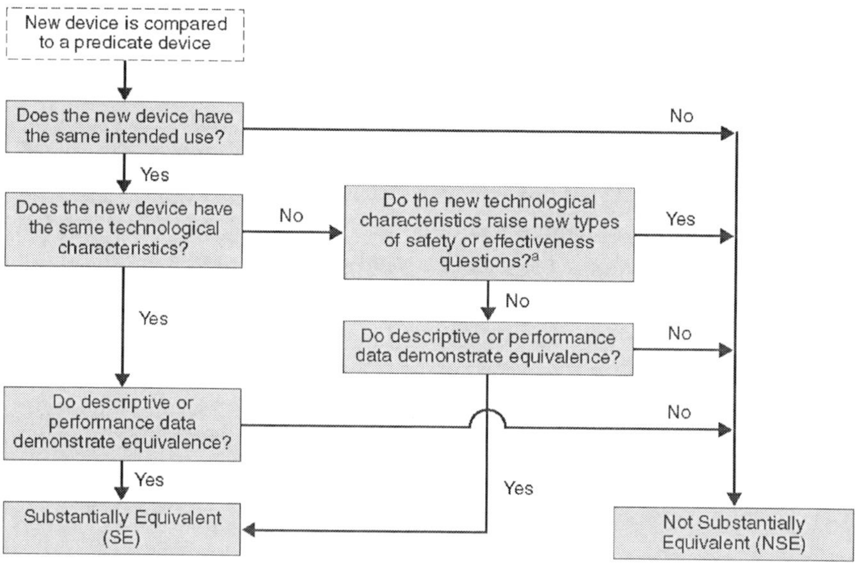

Source: GAO.

Notes: In cases where FDA determines that a new device has new technological characteristics that could not affect safety and effectiveness, the device may be determined SE if descriptive characteristics alone are precise enough to ensure equivalence. In cases where FDA determines that a new device has new technological characteristics that could affect safety and effectiveness, FDA requires performance data to demonstrate substantial equivalence. For cases in which descriptive or performance information is insufficient, FDA requests additional information.

[a] For devices with new technological characteristics, FDA first examines whether the new technological characteristics could affect safety or effectiveness.

Figure 2. FDA's 510(k) Decision-Making Process

Faster. FDA generally makes decisions on 510(k) submissions faster than it makes decisions on PMA submissions. FDA's fiscal year 2009 goal is to review and decide on 90 percent of 510(k) submissions within 90 days and 98 percent of them within 150 days. The comparable goal for PMAs is to review and decide upon 60 percent of original PMA submissions in 180 days and 90 percent of them within 295 days.[37]

Less expensive. The estimated cost to FDA for reviewing submissions is substantially lower for 510(k) submissions than for PMA submissions. For fiscal year 2005, for example, according to FDA the estimated average cost for the agency to review a 510(k) submission was about $18,200, while the estimate for a PMA submission was about $870,000. For the applicant, the standard fee provided to FDA at the time of submission is also significantly lower for a 510(k) submission than for a PMA submission. In fiscal year 2009, for example, the standard fee for 510(k) submissions is $3,693, while the standard fee for original PMA submissions is $200,725.[38]

Consumer advocates have raised questions regarding the number of devices, particularly class III devices, that are cleared through the 510(k) process and regarding the use of the 5 10(k) process to clear devices that may utilize new technologies that are different than those in the marketed devices to which they are compared. Officials of associations representing medical device manufacturers, however, have asserted that the 5 10(k) premarket review is an important tool for reviewing device submissions, saying that it is a rigorous process that gives FDA the flexibility to identify and request the information it needs to assess the safety and effectiveness of medical devices.

FDA USED THE 510(K) PROCESS TO REVIEW CLASS I AND II DEVICE SUBMISSIONS, AND USED BOTH THE 5 10(K) AND PMA PROCESSES TO REVIEW CLASS III DEVICE SUBMISSIONS

In fiscal years 2003 through 2007, FDA reviewed all submissions for class I and II devices through the 510(k) process, and reviewed submissions for some types of class III devices through the 510(k) process and others through the PMA process. Specifically, FDA reviewed all 13,199 submissions for class I and class II devices through the 510(k) process, clearing 11,935 (90 percent) of these submissions. FDA also reviewed 342 submissions for class III devices through the 510(k) process, clearing 228 (67 percent) of these submissions. In addition, the agency reviewed 217 original PMA submissions and 784 supplemental PMA submissions for class III devices and approved 78 percent and 85 percent, respectively, of these submissions. Although Congress envisioned that class III devices would be approved through the more stringent PMA process, we found that FDA has not published regulations requiring PMA submissions for some types of preamendment class III devices nor has it reclassified them. As a result, some types of class III devices have been cleared for the U.S. market through the 510(k) process.

Table 1 summarizes the FDA review decisions, by class of device, in fiscal years 2003 through 2007 for 510(k) and PMA submissions.

Table 1. FDA 510(k) and PMA Decisions by Class, Fiscal Years 2003 through 2007

Submission type	Device class	SE or approved (percentage of row)	NSE or denied (percentage of row)	Other decision[a] (percentage of row)	Total (percentage of row)
510(k)	Class I	1,265 (84)	40 (3)	204 (14)	1,509 (100)
	Class II	10,670 (91)	373 (3)	647 (6)	11,690 (100)
	Class III	228 (67)	100 (29)	14 (4)	342 (100)
	Other[b]	476 (33)	27 (2)	955 (66)	1,458 (100)
PMA					
Original	Class III	170 (78)	—[c]	47 (22)[c]	217 (100)
Supplemental[d]	Class III	664 (85)	—[c]	120 (15)[c]	784 (100)

Source: GAO analysis of FDA data.

Notes: Data represent 14,999 traditional and abbreviated 510(k) submissions, 217 original PMA submissions, and 784 supplemental PMA submissions for which FDA made review decisions in fiscal years 2003 through 2007. Percentages may not sum to 100 because of rounding.

[a] Other decisions include submissions that were withdrawn, were exempted by regulation, were not responsive to FDA's requests within a specified time frame, were forwarded to another FDA center (e.g., drugs or biologics), were duplicates, or were for products determined not to be devices.

[b] Other device class includes submissions for which a device class was not recorded in FDA's 510(k) database.

[c] According to FDA data, all PMA decisions during fiscal years 2003 through 2007 were approved or withdrawn. FDA did not deny approval of any PMA submissions during this period. According to FDA officials, when a PMA was seriously deficient, FDA issued a "not approvable" letter under 21 C.F.R. § 814.44(f) and placed the submission on hold. A company may withdraw a submission voluntarily. FDA also considers submissions to be withdrawn voluntarily if the applicant is unable to provide the information necessary to support approval within 180 days.

[d] Supplemental PMA submissions include 180-day (user-fee) and panel-track PMA supplements. The numbers in this row do not include other types of PMA supplements.

FDA Reviewed All Submissions for Class I and Class II Devices through the 510(k) Process

FDA reviewed all class I and class II device submissions in fiscal years 2003 through 2007 through the 510(k) process. As shown in table 2, FDA cleared approximately 9 out of every 10 of the 510(k) submissions for class I and class II devices for which FDA made review decisions during this time period.

Of the 10,670 510(k) submissions for class II devices that FDA cleared in fiscal years 2003 through 2007, FDA's databases identified one-quarter as being for devices that were implantable; were life sustaining; or presented significant risk to the health, safety, or welfare of a patient (see table 3). Of these characteristics, implantable was the most frequently identified characteristic. In terms of 510(k) submissions for class I devices, according to

FDA, none of the more than 1,200 510(k) submissions for class I devices that FDA cleared during the same time period were for devices that were implantable; were life sustaining; or presented significant risk to the health, safety, or welfare of a patient.

FDA Reviewed Submissions for Some Class III Devices Types through the 510(k) Process and Others through the PMA Process

In fiscal years 2003 through 2007, FDA reviewed submissions for some types of class III devices through the 510(k) process, and other types of class III devices through the PMA process. Specifically, FDA reviewed 342 submissions for new class III devices through the 510(k) process, determining 228 (67 percent) of these submissions to be SE to a predicate device.[39] During the same time period, FDA reviewed 217 original PMA submissions and 784 supplemental PMA submissions for class III devices and approved 78 percent and 85 percent of them, respectively. (See figure 3.)

FDA Has Not Issued Regulations Requiring PMA Submissions for Some Types of Class III Devices

Although Congress envisioned that class III devices would be approved through the more stringent PMA process, and the SMDA required that FDA establish a schedule for doing so, this process remains incomplete. The 228 class III submissions that FDA cleared through the 510(k) process in fiscal years 2003 through 2007 were allowed to undergo premarket review through the 510(k) process because they were for preamendment class III device types, or those substantially equivalent to them, for which FDA had not yet issued regulations either requiring PMA submissions or reclassifying them. These 228 5 10(k) submissions involved 24 device types (see table 4).[40] Of these types, 16 were included in one of the priority groups in FDA's 1994 strategy for reclassifying or requiring PMAs for class III device types, and in particular 4 device types—accounting for 39 of the 228 submissions—were among those that FDA identified as presenting an unreasonably high risk to public health.

The class III submissions FDA cleared through the 510(k) process were more likely than other 5 10(k) submissions to be for device types that were implantable; were life sustaining; or pose a significant risk to the health, safety, or welfare of a patient. Of the 228 510(k) submissions for class III devices that FDA cleared in fiscal years 2003 through 2007, FDA's databases flagged 66 percent as being for device types that are implantable, life sustaining, or of significant risk (see figure 4). This compares to no 510(k) submissions for class I devices and 25 percent of 510(k) submissions for class II devices.

Four of the 24 class III device types for which FDA cleared 510(k) submissions in fiscal years 2003 through 2007 have since been reclassified by FDA as class II device types.[41] Twenty of the 24 device types, however, may still be cleared through the 510(k) process.[42] Further, there are other preamendment class III device types that did not happen to have any 510(k) submissions cleared in fiscal years 2003 through 2007 that are also still eligible to be cleared through the 510(k) process.

FDA officials have acknowledged the importance of publishing regulations requiring PMA submissions or reclassifying preamendment class III device types. When asked for their time frame for doing so, the officials did not provide one. Rather, they responded that that the agency is committed to addressing this issue as resources and priorities permit.

Table 2. FDA Review Decisions for 510(k) Submissions for Class I and Class II Devices, by Fiscal Year (2003-2007)

Fiscal year	FDA decision			
	SE (percentage of row)	NSE (percentage of row)	Other decision[a] (percentage of row)	Total (percentage of row)
2003	2,519 (90)	72 (3)	215 (8)	2,806 (100)
2004	2,484 (92)	86 (3)	119 (4)	2,689 (100)
2005	2,395 (90)	89 (3)	164 (6)	2,648 (100)
2006	2,325 (91)	78 (3)	156 (6)	2,559 (100)
2007	2,212 (89)	88 (4)	197 (8)	2,497 (100)
Total	**11,935 (90)**	**413 (3)**	**851 (6)**	**13,199 (100)**

Source: GAO analysis of FDA data.

Note: Percentages may not sum to 100 because of rounding.

[a] Other decisions include submissions that were withdrawn, exempted by regulation, not responsive to FDA's requests within a specified time frame, forwarded to another FDA center or office, duplicates, or for products determined not to be devices or not actively regulated by FDA.

Table 3. 510(k) Submissions for Class I and Class II Devices Cleared in Fiscal Years 2003 through 2007

	Flag					
	Implantable only (percentage of row)	Life sustaining only (percentage of row)	Significant risk only (percentage of row)	More than one flag(percentage of row)	No flag (percentage of row)	Total (percentage of row)
Class I	0 (0)	0 (0)	0 (0)	0 (0)	1,265 (100)	**1,265 (100)**
Class II	1,957 (18)	266 (3)	159 (1)	235 (2)	8,053 (75)	**10,670 (100)**
Total	**1,957 (16)**	**266 (2)**	**159 (1)**	**235 (2)**	**9,318 (78)**	**11,935 (100)**

Source: GAO analysis of FDA data.

Note: Percentages may not sum to 100 because of rounding.

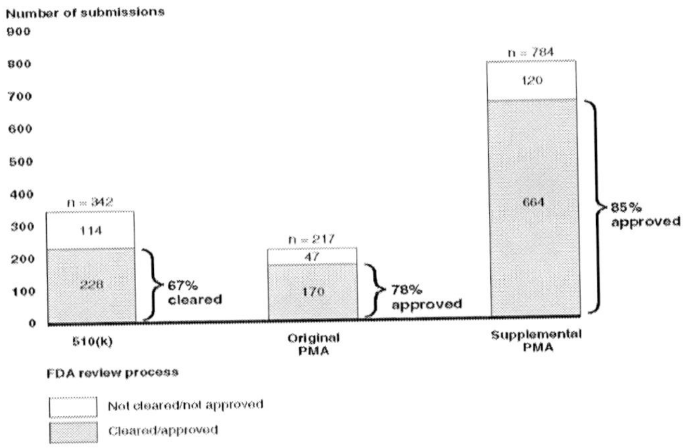

Source: GAO analysis of FDA data.

Notes: Figure represents FDA review decisions made between October 1, 2002, and September 30, 2007, for class III device submissions reviewed through the 510(k) and PMA processes. 510(k) includes traditional and abbreviated 510(k) submissions; *supplemental PMA* includes panel-track supplements and 180-day (user-fee) supplements.

Not cleared/not approved includes (1) for 510(k) submissions, those submissions FDA found to be NSE or withdrawn and (2) for PMA submissions, those submissions that were withdrawn. According to FDA data, all PMA decisions during fiscal years 2003 through 2007 were approved or withdrawn. FDA did not deny approval of any PMA submissions during this period. According to FDA officials, when a PMA is seriously deficient, FDA issues a "not approvable" letter and places the submission on hold. An applicant may then withdraw a submission voluntarily. FDA also considers submissions to be withdrawn voluntarily if the applicant is unable to provide the information necessary to support approval within 180 days.

Figure 3. Class III Device Submissions with FDA Review Decisions in Fiscal Years 2003 through 2007, by FDA Review Process and Review Decision

Table 4. Number of Submissions for Class III Devices Cleared through the 510(k) Process in Fiscal Years 2003 through 2007

Group	Number of device types	Number of submissions cleared in FYs 2003-2007	Examples
Included in a priority group in FDA's 1994 strategy	16	123	Certain types of hip joints, implanted blood access devices
Other[a]	8	105	Pedicle screws for certain types ofspinal surgeries, dental implants, automated external defibrillator
Total	**24**	**228**	

Source: GAO analysis of FDA data.

[a] Other includes device types for which FDA had already taken some action by 1994 (for example, FDA indicated that it had reclassification petitions pending for some device types in 1994) as well as new device types that FDA established after 1994 (for example, FDA issued a new regulation for a subset of one device type).

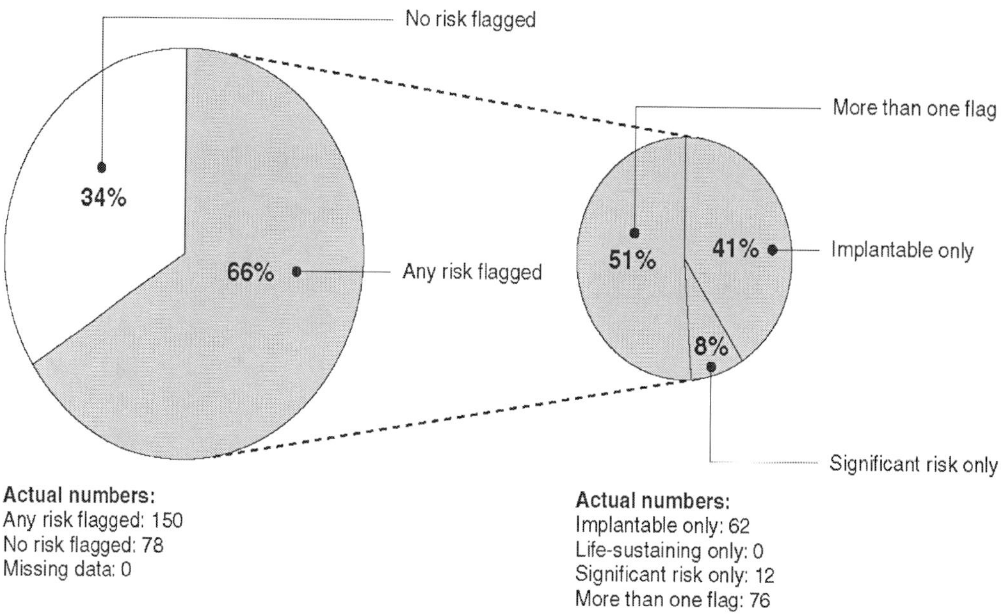

Source: GAO analysis of FDA data.

Notes: Figure represents data for 228 510(k) submissions for class III devices that FDA determined to be SE in fiscal years 2003 through 2007. FDA's database flagged 150 of these submissions as device types that were implantable; were life sustaining; presented significant risk to the health, safety, or welfare of a patient; or a combination of those flags.

Figure 4. Proportion of Cleared 510(k) Submissions for Class III Devices Flagged as Implantable, Life Sustaining, or of Significant Risk, Review Decisions Made in Fiscal Years 2003 through 2007

Relatively Few Class II and Class III 510(k) Submissions Had a New Intended Use or New Technological Characteristics

In our review of 510(k) submission files for which FDA reached a determination of SE or NSE in fiscal years 2005 through 2007, we found that FDA determined that relatively few devices had a new intended use or new technological characteristics. Overall, we found that FDA determined about 1 percent of class II and III submissions had a new intended use and about 15 percent had new technological characteristics.[43] For the 510(k) submissions that FDA cleared, FDA found that all of the devices had the same intended use as their predicate devices, and 86 percent also had the same technological characteristics. In contrast, of the 510(k) submissions that FDA determined to be NSE, more than half were for devices that had a new intended use or new technological characteristics.

Figure 5 shows the estimated percentage of 510(k) submissions reaching each step in the review process. See appendix V for additional information on FDA's decision-making process.

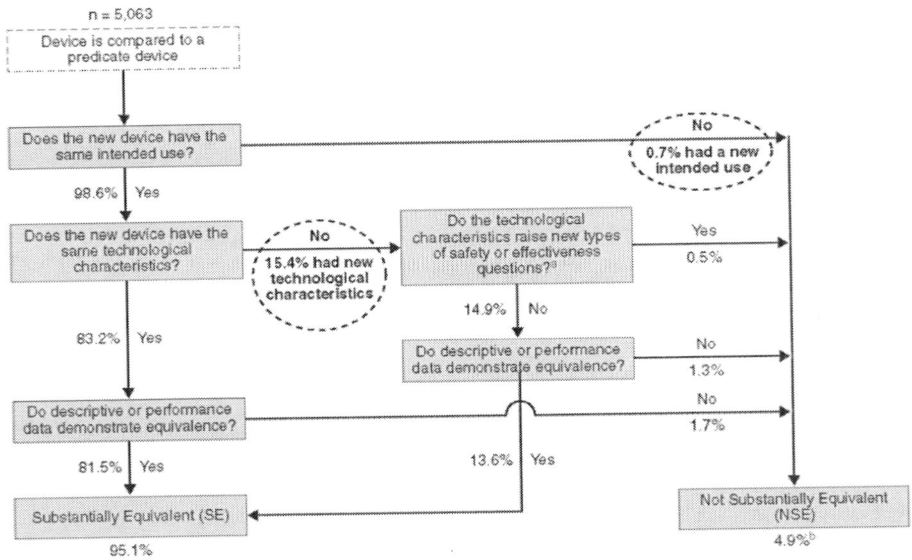

Source: GAO analysis of FDA files.

Notes: Estimates based on GAO review of all class III and a sample of class II 510(k) submissions. This figure includes data for 510(k) submissions for class II and class III devices that FDA determined to be SE and NSE in fiscal years 2005 through 2007. The sampling errors of the estimated percentages of 510(k) submissions reaching SE or NSE in FDA's decision-making process are within plus or minus 1 percentage point at the 95 percent confidence level.

In cases where FDA determines that a new device has new technological characteristics that could not affect safety and effectiveness, the device may be determined SE if descriptive characteristics alone are precise enough to ensure equivalence. In cases where FDA determines that a new device has new technological characteristics that could affect safety and effectiveness, FDA requires performance data to demonstrate substantial equivalence. For cases in which descriptive or performance information is insufficient, FDA requests additional information.

[a] For devices with new technological characteristics, FDA first examines whether the new technological characteristics could affect safety or effectiveness.

[b] Includes some submissions (0.6% of the 5,063 510(k) submissions) in which FDA made a determination of NSE but for which the determination path is not represented in this figure. Reasons that these cases were found NSE include the applicant failing to respond to an FDA data request and a PMA already being required for the device.

Figure 5. Projected Percentages of 510(k) Submissions for Class II and Class III Devices in Fiscal Years 2005 through 2007 Reaching Each Point in FDA's Decision-Making Process

All 510(k) Submissions That FDA Cleared Had the Same Intended Use and Most Had the Same Technological Characteristics as Predicate Devices

All 510(k) submissions for class II and class III devices that FDA cleared in fiscal years 2005 through 2007 had the same intended use and most had the same technological characteristics as predicate devices. In all 4,815 class II and class III submissions cleared through the 510(k) process during this time period, FDA determined that the new devices had the same intended use as their predicate devices. In 86 percent of these submissions, we found that FDA determined that the new devices also had the same technological characteristics as their predicate devices. (See figure 6.)

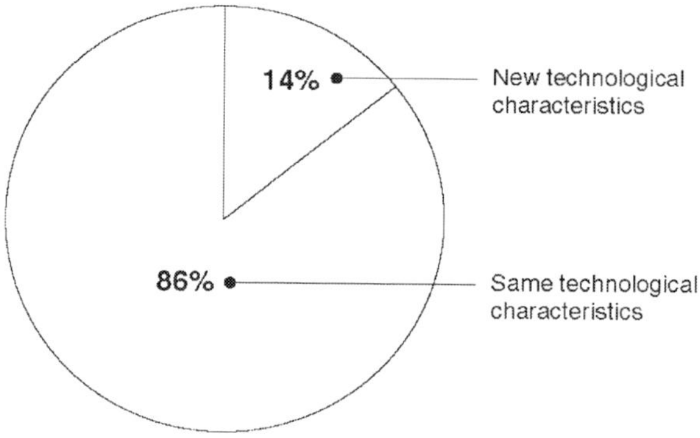

Source: GAO analysis of FDA files.

Notes: Data are estimated results for 4,815 submissions based on a sample of submissions for class II and class III devices cleared by FDA during fiscal years 2005 through 2007. The sampling errors of the estimated percentages in this chart are within plus or minus 5 percentage points at the 95 percent confidence level.

Figure 6. 510(k) Submissions Cleared in Fiscal Years 2005 through 2007, by Technological Characteristics

Table 5. Characteristics of Cleared 510(k) Submissions, Fiscal Years 2005 through 2007

Characteristics of cleared submissions	Class II (percentage)	Class III (percentage)	Total (percentage)
Same technological characteristics	4,052 (86)	75 (77)	**4,127 (86)**
New technological characteristics that could not affect safety or effectiveness	323 (7)	12 (12)	**335 (7)**
New technological characteristics that do not raise new types of safety or effectiveness questions	342 (7)	11 (11)	**353 (7)**
Total	**4,717 (100)**	**98 (100)**	**4,815 (100)**

Source: GAO analysis of FDA files.

Note: Data are estimated for 4,815 510(k) submissions based on a sample of submissions for class II and class III devices cleared by FDA in fiscal years 2005 through 2007. The sampling errors of the estimates of class II 510(k) submissions and total 510(k) submissions are within plus or minus 5 percentage points at the 95 percent confidence level.

In 14 percent of the class II and class III submissions cleared through the 510(k) process in fiscal years 2005 through 2007, FDA determined that the new device had new technological characteristics. For the cleared submissions with new technological characteristics, FDA determined, among other things, that either

1. the new technological characteristics could not affect safety or effectiveness—for example, FDA determined that software modifications to a defibrillator allowing physicians greater control over the device's CPR (cardiopulmonary resuscitation) settings could not affect the safety or effectiveness of the defibrillator—or
2. the new characteristics do not raise new types of safety or effectiveness questions—for example, FDA determined that a digital electrocardiograph did not raise new

types of effectiveness questions relative to the predicate device, an analog electrocardiograph.

Table 5 shows the distribution of cleared submissions by class and characteristics of the determination.

More Than Half of the 510(k) Submissions FDA Determined Not Substantially Equivalent Were for Devices That Had a New Intended Use or New Technological Characteristics

We found that of the 248 class II and III submissions that FDA determined to be NSE in fiscal years 2005 through 2007, slightly more than half

had a new intended use,
had a new technological characteristic that raised new types of safety or effectiveness questions, or
had a new technological characteristic that could affect safety or effectiveness and did not have performance data to demonstrate equivalence to the predicate device.

Table 6. Characteristics of 510(k) Submissions for Devices FDA Determined NSE in Fiscal Years 2005 through 2007

Characteristics	Class II (percentage)	Class III (percentage)	Total (percentage)
New intended use	15 (8)	22 (34)	**37 (15)**
New technological characteristics that raise new types of safety or effectiveness questions	19 (10)	22 (34)	**41 (17)**
New technological characteristics and insufficient performance data	42 (23)	7 (11)	**49 (20)**
Same technological characteristics, but insufficient performance data	88 (48)	1 (2)	**89 (36)**
Other[a]	19 (10)	13 (20)	**32 (13)**
Total	**183 (100)**	**65 (100)**	**248 (100)**

Source: GAO analysis of FDA files.

Notes: Data are estimated for 248 510(k) submissions for class II and class III devices that FDA determined NSE in fiscal years 2005 through 2007. The sampling errors of the estimates of class II 510(k) submissions and total 510(k) submissions are within plus or minus 10 percentage points at the 95 percent confidence level.

Percentages may not add to 100 because of rounding.

[a] Other includes 510(k) submissions for devices that were required to go through the PMA process, devices that did not have a predicate, and those that were determined to be NSE because of a lack of data early in the 510(k) process.

We also found that about one in every three 510(k) submissions FDA determined to be NSE had the same intended use and the same technological characteristics as the predicate device, but FDA determined the submissions NSE because of a lack of performance data. An additional 13 percent of submissions were determined NSE for other reasons, such as not providing adequate data early in the review or not having a predicate device (see table 6).

CONCLUSIONS

The 510(k) process plays a major role in FDA's oversight of medical devices. During fiscal years 2003 through 2007, FDA reviewed over 2,400 510(k) submissions annually and cleared about 90 percent of these submissions for the U.S. market. These included 228 cleared submissions for class III devices. In establishing device classes in 1976, Congress envisioned that all class III devices would eventually be required to undergo premarket review through the more stringent PMA process, which requires the manufacturer to provide evidence, which may include clinical data, providing reasonable assurance that the new device is safe and effective. However, certain preamendment class III device types may be reviewed through the 5 10(k) process until such time as FDA publishes regulations requiring them to go through the PMA process. In 1990 the SMDA directed FDA to take action on the remaining preamendment class III device types by reclassifying them to a lower class or requiring them to remain in class III and go through the PMA process, but we found that more than 14 years after FDA published its strategy and plans for doing so, a significant number of class III devices—including device types that FDA has identified as implantable; life sustaining; or posing a significant risk to the health, safety, or welfare of a patient—still enter the market through the less stringent 510(k) process.

FDA has stated that eventually all class III devices will require FDA approval through the PMA process and FDA officials reported that the agency is committed to addressing this issue, but the agency has not specified time frames for doing so. Without FDA action, the remaining preamendment class III device types—including device types that FDA identified in 1994 as presenting an unreasonably high risk to public health—may enter the U.S. market through FDA's less stringent premarket notification process.

RECOMMENDATION FOR EXECUTIVE ACTION

We are recommending that the Secretary of Health and Human Services direct the FDA Commissioner to expeditiously take steps to issue regulations for each class III device type currently allowed to enter the market through the 5 10(k) process. These steps should include issuing regulations to (1) reclassify each device type into class I or class II, or requiring it to remain in class III, and (2) for those device types remaining in class III, require approval for marketing through the PMA process.

AGENCY COMMENTS

We received comments on a draft of this report from HHS. (See app. VI.) The department commented that the draft report fairly and accurately describes FDA's 510(k) program and the department agreed with our conclusions and recommendation.

HHS agreed with our recommendation that FDA expeditiously take steps to reclassify or require PMAs for each class III device type currently allowed to enter the market through the 510(k) process, noting that since 1994 (when FDA announced it strategy to implement provisions of the Safe Medical Devices Act of 1990) FDA has called for PMAs or reclassified the majority of class III devices that did not require PMAs at that time. The department's comments, however, do not specify time frames in which FDA will address the remaining class III device types allowed to enter the market via the 510(k) process, stating instead that the agency is considering its legal and procedural options for completing this task as expeditiously as possible, consistent with available resources and competing time frames. Given that more than 3 decades have passed since Congress envisioned that all class III devices would eventually be required to undergo premarket review through the more stringent PMA process, it is imperative that FDA take immediate steps to address the remaining class III device types that may still enter the market through the less stringent 5 10(k) process by requiring PMAs for or reclassifying them.

The department also provided technical comments, which we incorporated as appropriate.

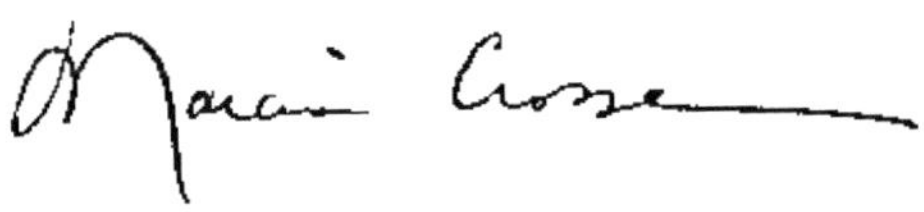

Marcia Crosse
Director, Health Care

APPENDIX I. SCOPE AND METHODOLOGY

To review the Food and Drug Administration's (FDA) use of the 510(k) and premarket approval (PMA) processes to review class I, II, and III device submissions in fiscal years 2003 through 2007, we used FDA's 510(k) and PMA databases. These databases contain information on device submissions,[44] including the name of the device, the FDA-assigned product code,[45] the status of the submission, and any FDA decisions related to the submission and the dates of those decisions. In both cases, we obtained and analyzed data on submissions for which FDA made a review decision in fiscal years 2003 through 2007.[46] We also used FDA's Device Nomenclature Management System to determine other attributes of the device types covered by the device submissions.

The 510(k) submissions we analyzed included traditional and abbreviated 510(k) submissions. We did not include special 510(k) submissions, which are requests for clearance of modifications to devices that have already been cleared through the 510(k) process (see table 7). The PMA submissions we analyzed included original PMA submissions and some supplemental PMA submissions. Specifically, we included supplemental PMA submissions that represented requests for approval for a significant change in a device: *panel-track supplements*, which are requests for approval for a significant change in design, performance, or use of a device for which clinical data are necessary to provide a reasonable assurance of safety and effectiveness; and *180-day* (*user-fee*) *supplements*, which are requests for approval for a significant change in components, materials, design, specification, software, color additives, or labeling. We did not include other types of PMA supplements, such as *real-time supplements*, which are requests for approval for a minor change to a device, such as a minor change in design, sterilization, software, or labeling.[47]

To assess the reliability of these data, we interviewed FDA officials knowledgeable about these databases, performed electronic testing for accuracy and completeness, and where applicable compared our results to aggregate information from other sources, such as published FDA reports and the FDA Web site. We determined that the data were sufficiently reliable for the purposes of this report.

In order to examine the extent to which FDA has determined that devices reviewed through the 510(k) process had new intended uses or new technological characteristics, we used FDA's 510(k) database to select and review a stratified random sample of class II and all class III 510(k) submission files from fiscal years 2005 through 2007. See table 7 for the scope of our file review.

All 163 class III submissions that met the inclusion criteria were included in the sample. The 296 class II cases included in the sample constituted a random sample of the 4,900 class II submissions that met the inclusion criteria. The class II submissions included in the sample were stratified by decision, meaning that class II submissions determined not substantially equivalent (NSE) were oversampled so that the results could be generalizable to the universe of all class II submissions, to class II submissions determined NSE, or to class II submissions determined substantially equivalent (SE). The sample contained a total of 459 submissions. See tables 8 and 9 for the number of submissions by fiscal year, class, and decision.

We conducted our file review in June 2008. We collected data primarily from the FDA reviewer memo, which contained information concerning the steps FDA took to reach its determination of SE or NSE. This information included the incremental decisions FDA made concerning the use and technological characteristics of the new device, and in sum, defined the path through an FDA decision tree the reviewer took to reach a determination of SE or NSE. See figures 7 and 8 for detailed and simplified versions, respectively, of FDA's decision tree. We recorded the individual decisions made in each case, and analyzed the results with respect to the path the FDA reviewer took to reach the final determination of SE or NSE.

In the 10 cases where we could not determine the steps FDA took to reach its determination during our file review, we requested additional information from FDA officials. Officials from the Office of Device Evaluation in FDA's Center for Devices and Radiological Health reviewed the files in question and provided us with the information we requested.

To assess the reliability of these data, we compared our results with information from FDA's 510(k) database and Device Nomenclature Management System. In addition, FDA officials stated that the data in the files were accurate and reliable and provided input in the development of our data collection instrument.

Table 7. Scope of File Review by 510(k) Submission Type, Review Decision, and FDA Office or Center

Characteristic of 510(k) submission	Included in file review?	Reason
Submission type		
Traditional	Yes	Traditional 510(k) submissions are the conventional 510(k) submission type used to clear new devices for market. Traditional submissions constituted the majority of 510(k) submissions made to FDA during the time of our review.
Abbreviated	Yes	Abbreviated 510(k) submissions are a streamlined version of the traditional 510(k) process. In an abbreviated 510(k) submitssion, applicants use guidance documents, special controls, or performance standards to assess and then report on the performance of their new device to expedite review.
Special	No	Special 510(k) submissions are submitted for a modification to a device that has been cleared through the 510(k) process. We excluded them from our review because this type of submission is only used for modifications to a device which has already cleared the 510(k) process.
Review decision		
Substantially equivalent (SE)	Yes	The submissions completed the 510(k) review process and were cleared for market.
Not substantially equivalent (NSE)	Yes	The submissions completed the 510(k) review process and were not cleared for market.
Withdrawn	No	Withdrawn submissions did not complete the 510(k) review process.
Deleted	No	Deleted submissions did not complete the 510(k) review process.
FDA office or center		
Center for Devices and Radiological Health, Office of Device Evaluation	Yes	This office administers the 510(k), PMA, Humanitarian Device Exemption, and Investigational Device Exemption progr-ams. It processes the majority of 510(k) submissions each year: for example, in FY 2007, it processed 85 percent of all 510(k) submissions.
Center for Devices and Radiological Health, Office of In Vitro Diagnostic Device Evaluation and Safety	No	This office oversees the regulation of devices such as in-home and laboratory diagnostic tests, and processes relatively few 510(k) submissions each year. In FY 2007, it processed 13 percent of all 510(k) submissions.
Center for Biologics Evaluation and Research	No	This office oversees devices such as those used for licensed blood collection and processing, and processes relatively few 510(k) submissions each year. In FY 2007, it processed 2 percent of all 510(k) submissions.

Source: GAO.

Note: The scope of the file review also excluded de novo submissions, which are submissions for first-of-a-kind devices lacking a legally marketed predicate. See 21 U.S.C. § 360c(f)(2).

Table 8. Cases Reviewed, by Fiscal Year

Fiscal year	Count	Percentage
2005	167	36
2006	141	31
2007	151	33
Total	459	100

Source: GAO.

Table 9. Cases Reviewed, by Class and SE/NSE Determination

FDA decision	Class II	Class III	Total
SE	195	102	297
NSE	101	61	162
Total	296	163	459

Source: GAO.

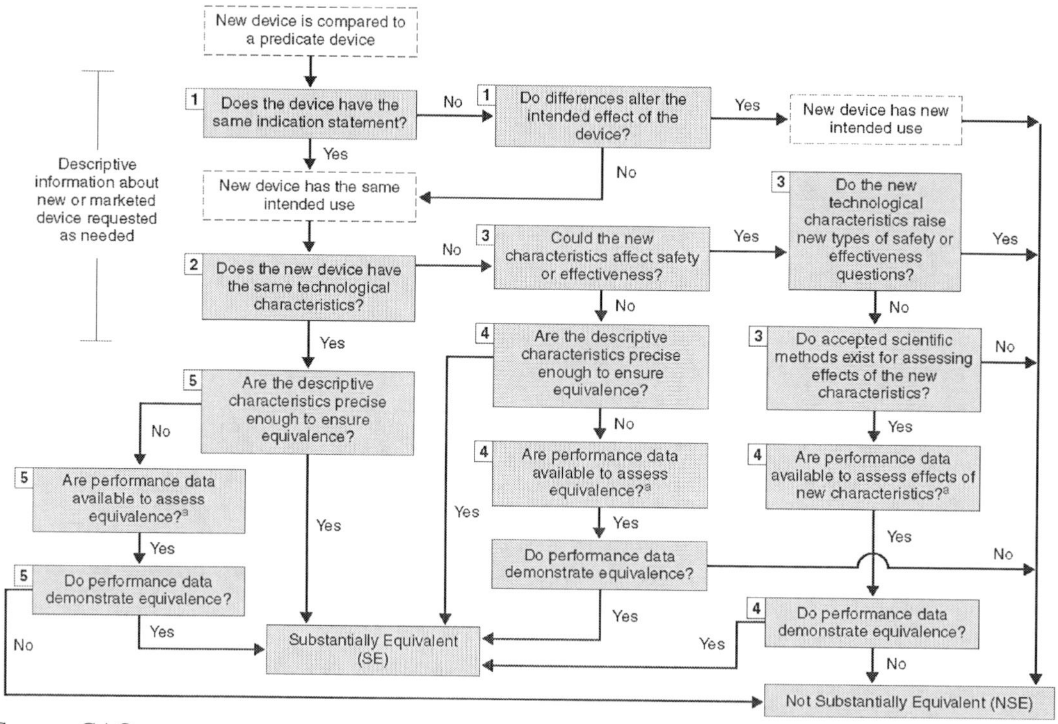

Source: GAO.

Notes: Numbered boxes correspond to numbered boxes on the simplified FDA decision-making process in figure 8.

[a] Data may be in the 510(k), other 51 0(k)s, the center's classification files, or the literature. In cases where FDA determines that performance data are not available, FDA requests data from the applicant.

Figure 7. Detailed Version of FDA's 510(k) Decision-Making Process

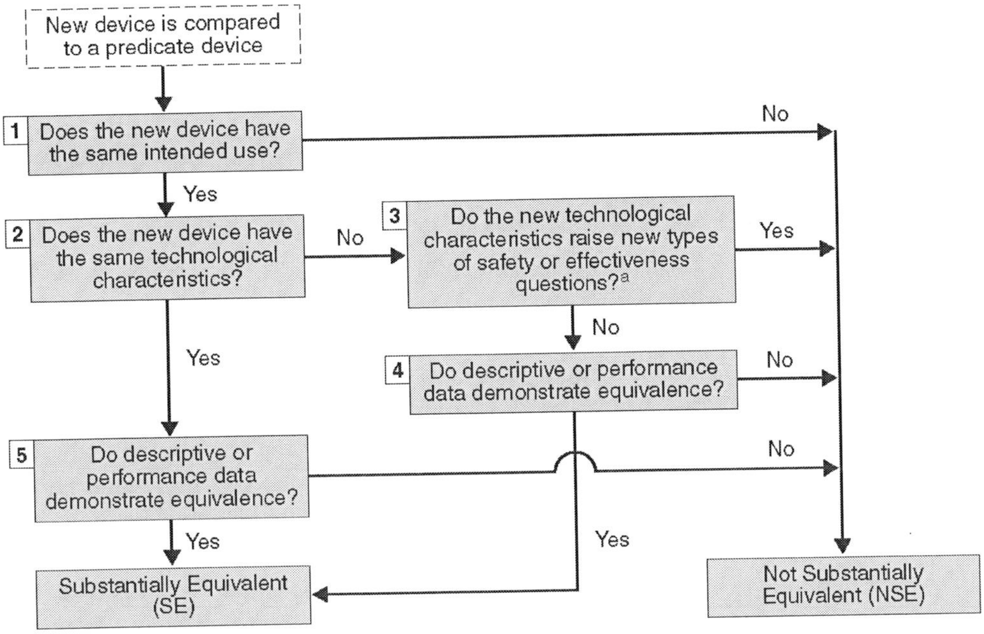

Source: GAO.

Notes: Numbered boxes correspond to numbered boxes on the detailed decision tree in figure 7.

In cases where FDA determines that a new device has new technological characteristics that could not affect safety and effectiveness, the device may be determined SE if descriptive characteristics alone are precise enough to ensure equivalence. If not, FDA will look at performance data. In cases where FDA determines that a new device has new technological characteristics that could affect safety and effectiveness, FDA requires performance data to demonstrate substantial equivalence. For cases in which descriptive or performance information is insufficient, FDA requests additional information.

[a] For devices with new technological characteristics, FDA first examines whether the new technological characteristics could affect safety or effectiveness.

Figure 8. Simplified Version of FDA's 510(k) Decision-Making Process

In addition to our data analysis, we reviewed relevant laws and regulations concerning the premarket review process. We also interviewed FDA officials from the FDA centers and offices that process device submissions (Center for Biologics Evaluation and Research, Office of Device Evaluation, and Office of In Vitro Diagnostic Device Evaluation and Safety). Finally, we interviewed representatives from professional associations representing device manufacturers (the Advanced Medical Technology Association, the ECRI Institute, the Medical Device Manufacturers Association, and the Medical Imaging and Technology Alliance) and consumer advocates (the National Research Center for Women & Families and Public Citizen).

We conducted this performance audit from March 2008 to January 2009 in accordance with generally accepted government auditing standards. Those standards require that we plan and perform the audit to obtain sufficient, appropriate evidence to provide a reasonable basis for our findings and conclusions based on our audit objectives. Wc believe that the evidence obtained provides a reasonable basis for our findings and conclusions based on our audit objectives.

APPENDIX II. THIRD-PARTY REVIEW OF 510(K) SUBMISSIONS

The FDA Modernization Act of 1997 directed FDA to accredit third parties (called accredited persons) in the private sector to conduct the initial review of 510(k) submissions for low- to moderate-risk devices.[48] Under FDA's Accredited Persons Program, device manufacturers may contract with accredited organizations (third parties)[49] to review certain 510(k) submissions for a negotiated fee.[50] The third party uses the same statutory and regulatory criteria as FDA to determine substantial equivalence, documents its review and recommendation, and forwards the 5 10(k) submission and documentation to FDA's Center for Devices and Radiological Health. At the center, a third-party 510(k) submission is assessed by an FDA supervisor, who may accept or change the substantial equivalence recommendation of the third party. After completing the supervisory assessment, FDA issues a letter to the 510(k) applicant via the third-party reviewer with a final determination on the 510(k) submission. During the third-party review, the FDA supervisor can request additional information from the third party and the third party can request additional information from the 510(k) applicant.

FDA expanded the program to include more than 670 class I and class II device types to be eligible for 510(k) review by a third party.[51] These include device types for diagnostic ultrasound systems, computed tomography X-ray systems, and surgical lasers. However, not all of the accredited third parties are authorized to review all device types eligible for third-party review. For example, in October 2008 FDA's Web site listed 7 of 11 accredited third parties as authorized to review 510(k) submissions for hearing aids.

Device types that are not eligible for third-party review include all class III devices; class II devices intended to be permanently implantable, life sustaining, or life supporting; and class II devices requiring clinical data to support their 510(k) clearance.[52] During our review of FDA's 510(k) database, we found three instances of 510(k) submissions in which class II devices that were life sustaining were cleared for market through the third-party review program during fiscal years 2003 through 2007. FDA officials explained that about five life-sustaining, class II device types, hemodialysis devices, had inadvertently been added to the list of devices eligible for third-party review when the list was expanded in 2001, and that in May 2003, FDA removed the life-sustaining class II device types from the list of devices eligible for third-party review on FDA's Web site. The FDA officials said that while the three 510(k) submissions for class II life- sustaining device submissions had been submitted through the third-party review program, FDA also conducted its own review of the three 510(k) submissions before they were cleared for marketing.

During fiscal years 2003 through 2007, FDA reviewed and made final determinations on 1,082 third-party 510(k) submissions (see table 10). According to FDA, the number of third-party submissions increased as the result of (1) increased familiarity with the third-party review program among potential applicants, (2) the increase in the number of device types eligible for the program, and (3) less financial disincentives to use the third-party review program as FDA instituted device user fees.[53] An FDA official familiar with the program stated that the third-party review program may be more attractive to device manufacturers because third- party review 510(k) submissions are processed faster than traditional 510(k) submissions. The official noted, however, that as FDA's review of traditional 510(k) submissions becomes more efficient, the advantages of the third-party review program in terms of timeliness may diminish, which could lead to fewer third-party review 510(k) submissions.[54]

Table 11 shows the third-party review 510(k) submissions by medical specialty.

Table 10. Third-Party Review 510(k) Submissions with FDA Decisions, Fiscal Years 2003 through 2007 FDA decision

	FDA decision		
Fiscal year	**SE (percentage)**	**NSE (percentage)**	**Total (percentage)**
2003	157 (15)	2 (10)	**159 (15)**
2004	227 (21)	9 (43)	**236 (22)**
2005	226 (21)	3 (14)	**229 (21)**
2006	242 (23)	6 (29)	**248 (23)**
2007	209 (20)	1 (5)	**210 (19)**
Total	**1,061 (100)**	**21 (100)**	**1,082 (100)**

Source: GAO analysis of FDA data.

Note: Percentages may not sum to 100 because of rounding.

Table 11. Third-Party Review 510(k) Submissions by Medical Specialty, Fiscal Years 2003 through 2007

Medical specialty	Frequency	Percentage
Radiology	411	38.7
General and plastic surgery	120	11.3
Cardiovascular	116	10.9
General hospital	98	9.2
Dental	52	4.9
Gastroenterology and urology	49	4.6
Anesthesiology	45	4.2
Neurology	45	4.2
Physical medicine	43	4.1
Ophthalmic	25	2.4
Obstetrics and gynecology	22	2.1
Clinical chemistry	13	1.2
Ear, nose, and throat	7	0.7
Clinical toxicology	4	0.4
Microbiology	4	0.4
Hematology	3	0.3
Orthopedic	3	0.3
Immunology	1	0.1
Total	**1,061**	**100**

Source: GAO analysis of FDA data.

Note: Percentages may not sum to 100 because of rounding.

Appendix III. FDA's Implementation of Safe Medical Devices Act Provisions

The Safe Medical Devices Act of 1990 (SMDA) amended the definition of class II devices[55] and required FDA, for each preamendment class III device type and before December 1, 1995, to (1) order manufacturers to submit information on safety and effectiveness to FDA and (2) publish proposed and final regulations to reclassify each device type into class II or class I or to require it to remain in class III. For those devices for which FDA published a regulation requiring the device to remain in class III, the SMDA further directed FDA to, as promptly as reasonably achievable but not later than 12 months after the effective date of the regulation requiring the device to remain in class III, establish a schedule for the promulgation of regulations requiring the submission of PMAs.

In an April 19, 1994, memorandum from the Acting Director of the FDA Center for Devices and Radiological Health's Office of Device Evaluation, FDA outlined its strategy for implementation of the SMDA. Specifically, FDA grouped 117 preamendment class III device types for which FDA had not yet initiated any action to require the submission of PMAs into three groups and prioritized the devices to facilitate the SMDA activities. (See table 12.) The agency's proposed strategy established a plan for beginning to address the class III device types that were continuing to be reviewed through the 510(k) process, but did not establish completion dates for doing so.

Table 12. FDA Groupings and Time Frames for Implementation of SMDA Provisions for Class III Device Types in 1994 and Status as of October 2008

Group 3 (device types designated high priority)	
Number of device types	15
Description	Group 3 contains devices that were not considered candidates for reclassify-cation and thatFDA believed were in commercial distribution and would require submission of PMAs in the near future. The high-priority subgroup of group 3 contains devices FDA determined presented an unreasonably high risk to public health because significant issues of safety, effectiveness, or both were not being resolved or, to the best of FDA's knowledge, had little probability ofbeing resolved.
Examples	Certain types of hip joints and shoulder joints, ultrasound and muscle stimulator.
Planned schedule	FDA planned to publish proposed rules related to these 15 device types by 1996. In its 1994 strategy memorandum, FDA noted that the timetable for publication of each final rule would be based upon specific data needs, comments received, and the existence, if any, of any petitions to reclassify the devices that FDA needed to review.
Status as of October 2008	Of the 15 device types designated high priority in group 3, 5 were reclassified, 6 now require PMAs, and 4 may still be cleared through the 510(k) process.
Number of device types	27

Description	Group 3 contains devices that were not considered candidates for reclassify-ication and thatFDA believed were in commercial distribution and would require submission of PMAs in the near future. The devices in group 3 that were not designated high priority were not considered candidates for reclassification, but FDA planned to assess whether these devices should be moved to group 2. FDA stated that the continued marketing of these group 3 devices did not present as great a risk to the public health, in light of FDA's knowledge and experience with the devices, as the device types designated high priority.
Examples	External pacemaker pulse generator, stairclimbing wheelchair.
Planned schedule	FDA planned to pursue the same course of evaluation and prioritization as used for group 2 device types.
Status as of October 2008	Of the 27 other device types in group 3 that were not designated high priority, 13 were reclassified, 7 now require PMAs, and 7 may still be cleared through the 510(k) process.
Group 2	
Number of device types	31
Description	Group 2 contains devices that FDA believed had a high potential for reclassification into class II and for which existing questions of safety, effectiveness, or both had been or could be answered by information already obtained or being obtained by manufacturers. According to FDA, the SMDA-modified definition of class II devices together with increased experience with these device types might provide grounds for reclassification of group 2 devices.
Examples	Tweezer-type epilator, cardiovascular permanent pacemaker electrodes, implanted blood access device.
Group 3 (device types designated high priority)	
Planned schedule	FDA planned to issue an order requiring manufacturers to submit all safety and effectiveness information available or known to them, including adverse information, for allgroup 2 device types, to complete a review and evalua-tion of this safety and effectiveness information, and to proceed with rule making to reclassify these device types or retain them in class III by 1998. The 1994 memorandum did not specify any dates for publicationof final regulations reclassifying devices or requiring them to remain in class III.
Status as of October 2008	Of the 31 device types in group 2, 23 were reclassified, 1 now requires a PMA, and 7 may still be cleared through the 510(k) process (this includes 1 case in which the device type was reclassified for some purposes but remains class III for others).
Group 1	
Number of device types	44
Description	Group 1 contains device types that FDA identified as having fallen into disuse or limited use. FDA determined that these device types raise signify-cant questions of safety, effectiveness, or both but are rarely in current use. FDA believed that rule making requiring PMAs for these device types would be unlikely to result in viable PMAs or reclassification petitions.
Examples	Catheter balloon repair kit; certain types of hip joints, finger joints, and shoulder joints.

Table 12. (continued)

Group 1	
Planned schedule	FDA planned to publish one proposed regulation in 1994 requiring PMAs for all group 1 devices. The 1994 memorandum did not specify any dates for publication of final regulations.
Status as of October 2008	Of the 44 device types in group 1, 4 were reclassified, 39 now require PMAs, and 1 may still be cleared through the 510(k) process.
All groups	
Number of device types	117
Status as of October 2008	Of the 117 device types contained in FDA's strategy document, 45 have been reclassified,53 now require PMAs, and 19 may still be cleared through the 510(k) process.

Source: GAO.

Note: In addition, the 1994 memorandum listed additional device types for which some action had been taken toward reclassification or requiring PMA submissions. For example, the memorandum listed device types, including endosseous (dental) implants, with reclassification petitions pending.

As of October 2008, FDA had reclassified 45 device types and published regulations requiring PMAs for 53 device types. Therefore, of the 117 preamendment class III device types covered by FDA's strategy, 19 device types remain in class III and may be cleared through the 510(k) process.[56] Four of those 19 device types are types that FDA had placed in group 3 and designated high priority—that is, they are device types that FDA had determined to present an unreasonably high risk to public health because significant issues of safety or effectiveness were not being resolved or, to the best of FDA's knowledge, had little probability of being resolved.

Appendix IV. Additional Information on 510(k) Submissions for Class III Devices Reviewed by FDA

This appendix summarizes the results from GAO analysis of FDA's data for class III 510(k) submissions with FDA review decisions in fiscal years 2003 through 2007. The following tables show FDA's final decisions for submissions for class III devices for each fiscal year through the 510(k) process (table 13); the primary medical specialties for submissions for class III devices cleared through the 510(k) process (table 14); and a detailed list of all device types covered by the class III devices cleared through the 510(k) process, including the status of these device types as of October 2008 (table 15).

Table 13. FDA Review Decisions for Class III 510(k) Submissions by Fiscal Year, Fiscal Years 2003 through 2007

	FDA Decision			
Fiscal Year	**SE (percentage of row)**	**NSE (percentage of row)**	**Other[a] (percentage of row)**	**Total (percentage of row)**
2003	58 (80)	12 (16)	3 (4)	**73 (100)**
2004	68 (80)	13 (15)	4 (5)	**85 (100)**
2005	31 (52)	27 (45)	2 (3)	**60 (100)**
2006	32 (50)	31 (48)	1 (2)	**64 (100)**
2007	39 (65)	17 (28)	4 (7)	**60 (100)**
Total	**228 (67)**	**100 (29)**	**14 (4)**	**342 (100)**

Source: GAO analysis of FDA data.

[a] Other decisions include submissions that were withdrawn, exempted by regulation, not responsive to FDA's requests within a specified time frame, forwarded to another FDA center or office, duplicates, determined not to be a device, or not actively regulated by FDA.

Table 14. Primary Medical Specialties of Class III 510(k) Submissions Cleared in Fiscal Years 2003 through 2007

Medical specialty	Frequency	Percentage
Cardiovascular	64	28
Orthopedic	54	24
Gastroenterology and urology	36	16
Dental	31	14
Physical medicine	19	8
Neurology	14	6
Microbiology	7	3
General and plastic surgery	2	1
Obstetrics and gynecology	1	1
Total	**228**	**100**

Source: GAO analysis of FDA data.

Note: Totals may not sum to 100 because of rounding.

Table 15. Device Types with Class III 510(k) Submissions Cleared in Fiscal Years 2003 through 2007 and Their Status as of October 2008

Device type (regulation number)	Number of submissions cleared in FYs 2003-2007	Actions taken as of October 2008
Device types included in group 3 and designated high priority in FDA's 1994 strategy[a]		
Iontophoresis device[b] (21 C.F.R. § 890.5525(b))	18	FDA published a notice of intent to reclassify this device type in 2000. FDA has not issued a regulation reclassifying or requiring PMA submissions for this device type. It remains a class III type that may be cleared through the 510(k) process.

Table 15. (continued)

Device type (regulation number)	Number of submissions cleared in FYs 2003-2007	Actions taken as of October 2008
Device types included in group 3 and designated high priority in FDA's 1994 strategy[a]		
Hip joint metal/ Metal semiconstra-ined, with an unce-mented acetabular component, prosthe-sis (21 C.F.R. § 888.3330)	18	FDA rejected one petition to reclassify this device type in 2002 and received another classification peti-tion in 2005. According toFDA officials, the agency is reviewing the reclassification petitionthat it received in 2005. While it is doing so, this remains a class III device type that may be cleared through the 510(k) process.
Hip joint metal/ metal semi-constrai-ned, with a cemented acetabular component, prosthesis (21 C.F.R. § 888.3320)	2	FDA rejected one petition to reclassify this device type in 2002 and received another classification petition in 2005. According toFDA officials, the agency is reviewing the petition that it receivedin 2005. While it is doing so, this remains a class III device type that may be cleared through the 510(k) process.
Shortwave diathermy[c] (21 C.F.R. § 890.5290)	1	FDA requested that manufacturers submit safety and effectiveness information by August 14, 1997. FDA has not issued a regulation reclassifying or requiring PMA submissions for this device type. It remains a class III type that may be cleared through the 510(k) process.
Neurovascular emb-olization device[d](21 C.F.R. § 882.5950)	11	FDA reclassified this device type to class II effective January 28, 2005.
External counter-pulsating device (21 C.F.R. § 870.5225)	9	FDA requested that manufacturers submit safety and effectiveness information by February 14, 1997. FDA has not issued a regulation reclassifying or requiring PMA submissions for this device type. It remains a class III type that may be cleared through the 510(k) process.
Arrythmia detector and alarm (21 C.F.R. § 870.1025)	7	FDA reclassified this device type to class II effective November 28, 2003.
Vascular emboli-zation device[d](21 C.F.R. § 870.3300)	4	FDA reclassified this device type to class II effective January 28, 2005.
Intra-aortic balloon and control system (21 C.F.R. § 870.3535)	2	FDA requested that manufacturers submit safety and effectiveness information by August 14, 1997. FDA has not issued a regulation reclassifying or requiring PMA submissions for this device type. It remains a class III type that may be cleared through the 510(k) process.
Sorbent hemoper-fusion system (21 C.F.R. § 876.5870)	1	FDA requested that manufacturers submit safety and effectiveness information by February 14, 1998. FDA has not issued a regulation reclassifying or requiring PMA submissions for this device type. It remains a class III type that may be cleared through the 510(k) process.
External pacemaker pulse generator(21	1	FDA that requested manufacturers submit safety and effectiveness information by August 14, 1997. FDA has

C.F.R. § 870.3600)		not issued a regulation reclassifying or requiring PMA submissions for this device type. It remains a class III type that may be cleared through the 510(k) process.
Blood access device (implanted) (21 C.F.R. § 876.5540(b)(1))	35	FDA requested that manufacturers submit safety and effectiveness information by August 14, 1998. FDA has not issued a regulation reclassifying or requiring PMA submissions for this device type. It remains a class III type that may be cleared through the 510(k) process.
Herpes simplex virus serological assays[d] (21 C.F.R. § 866.3305)	7	FDA reclassified this device type to class II for type 1 and/or type 2 serological assays effective May 3, 2007; all other assays remain class III and may be cleared through the 510(k) process. According to FDA, the seven class III 510(k) submissions for herpes simplex virus serological assays cleared in fiscal years 2003 through 2007 were for type 1 and/or type 2 serological assays.
External cardiac compressor (21 C.F.R. § 870.5200)	4	FDA requested that manufacturers submit safety and effectiveness information by August 14, 1998. FDA has not issued a regulation reclassifying or requiring PMA submissions for this device type. It remains a class III type that may be cleared through the 510(k) process.
Topical oxygen chamber for extre-mities (21 C.F.R. § 878.5650)	2	FDA requested that manufacturers submit safety and effectiveness information by August 14, 1997; FDA published a proposal to reclassify in 2006. FDA has not issued a regulation reclassifying or requiring PMA submissions for this device type. It remains a class III type that may be cleared through the 510(k) process.
Cardiovascular pacemaker electr-odes (permanent) (21 C.F.R. § 870.3680)	1	FDA requested that manufacturers submit safety and effectiveness information by August 14, 1997. FDA has not issued a regulation reclassifying or requiring PMA submissions for this device type. It remains a class III type that may be cleared through the 510(k) process.
Other[e]		
Pedicle screw spinal system[f] (21 C.F.R. § 888.3070(b)(2))	34	In 2001, FDA stated that it intended to initiate the call for PMAs for the device when intended for certain uses in a future *FederalRegister*notice. FDA has not issued a regulation reclassifying or requiring PMA submissions for this device type. It remains a class III type that may be cleared through the 510(k) process.
Automated external defibrillator (21 C.F.R. § 870.5310)	30	In 2003, FDA began to regulate automated external defibrillators separately from arrhythmia detectors and alarms; at that time, theagency published a notice of intent to initiate a proceeding to reclassify. FDA has not issued a regulation reclassifying or requiring PMA submissions for this device type. It remains a class III type that may be cleared through the 510(k) process.
Endosseous dental implant (blade form) (21 C.F.R. § 872.3640(b)(2))	26	FDA reclassified this device type to class II for root-form endosseous dental implants effective June 11, 2004; blade-form endosseous dental implants remain class III and may be clearedthrough the 510(k) process.

Table 15. (continued)

Device type (regulation number)	Number of submissions cleared in FYs 2003-2007	Actions taken as of October 2008
Device types included in group 3 and designated high priority in FDA's 1994 strategy[a]		
Endosseous dental implant abutment (21 C.F.R. § 872.3630)	4	FDA reclassified this device type to class II effective June 11, 2004.
Nonroller-type cardiopulmonary bypass blood pump (21 C.F.R. § 870.4360)	5	FDA had published a proposal to reclassify the device in 1993 and withdrew that proposal in 2004. FDA has not issued a regulation reclassifying or requiring PMA submissions for this device type. It remains a class III type that may be cleared through the 510(k) process.
Cranial electrotherapy stimulator (21 C.F.R. § 882.5800)	3	FDA had required PMA submissions for this device type in 1995 but revoked that regulation in 1997. FDA requested safety and effectiveness information from manufacturers in 1997. FDA has not issued a regulation reclassifying or requiring PMA submissions for this device type. It remains a class III type that may be cleared through the 510(k) process.
Mandibular condyle prosthesis (temporary)[g] (21 C.F.R. § 872.3960)	1	FDA amended the regulation in 1998 stating that no effective date had been established for the submission of PMAs for the implanted version of the device used for temporary reconstruction. In the applicable *Federal Register* notice, FDA added that at a later date, it would propose reclassifying from class III to class II the generic type of temporary mandibular condyle prosthesis intended for temporary reconstruction following surgical ablation of malignant and benign tumors. FDA has not issued a regulation reclassifying or requiring PMA submissions for this device type. It remains a class III type that may be cleared through the 510(k) process.
Pericardial patch	2	According to agency officials, FDA is in the process of determining how to address the situation under which FDA cleared two submissions for this type of class III device through the 510(k) process).

Source: GAO.

Notes: No submissions with device types included in group 1 of FDA's 1994 strategy were cleared in fiscal years 2003 through 2007. Generally, the name of the device type is the title of the relevant provision in the 2008 edition of title 21 of the *Code of Federal Regulations*.

[a] For a detailed description of the device types covered by FDA's 1994 strategy, see app. III.

[b] For uses other than (1) the diagnosis of cystic fibrosis or (2) those indicated on the label of the drug used with the device if the label includes adequate directions for the device's use with the drug.

[c] For uses other than (1) the treatment of malignancies or (2) the generation of deep heat within body tissues to treat conditions such as pain, muscle spasms, and joint contractures.

[d] During the period of our review, FDA renamed these devices: the neurovascular embolization device, vascular embolization device, and herpes simplex virus serological assays were previously know as the artificial embolization device, arterial embolization device, and herpes simplex virus serological reagents, respectively.

[e] Other includes device types for which FDA had already taken some action by 1994 (for example, FDA indicated that it had reclassification petitions pending for some device types in 1994) as well as new device types that FDA established after 1994 (for example, FDA added a regulation for a subset of one device type).

[f] When intended to provide immobilization and stabilization of spinal segments in the thoracic, lumbar, and sacral spine as an adjunct to fusion in the treatment of degenerative disc disease and spondylolisthesis other than either severe spondylolisthesis (grades 3 and 4) at L5-S1 or degenerative spondylolisthesis with objective evidence of a neurologic impairment.

[g] In 1998 FDA issued a regulation requiring PMAs for mandibular condyle prostheses intended for permanent reconstruction.

Appendix V. FDA's 510(k) Decision-Making Process

This appendix presents the additional information from GAO analysis of FDA's 5 10(k) submission files for which FDA reached a determination of SE or NSE in fiscal years 2005 through 2007. The following figures show FDA's detailed decision-making process for class II and class III submissions (figure 9); the decision-making process for class II devices alone (figure 10); and the decision-making process for class III devices alone (figure 11).

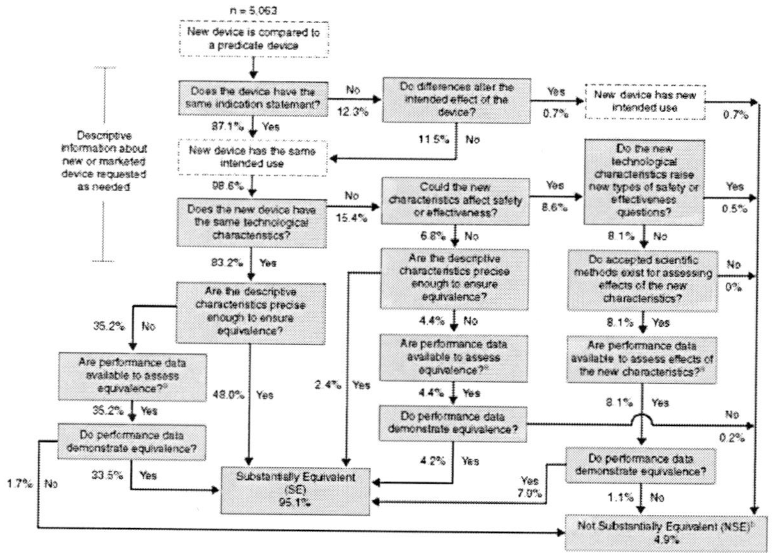

Source: GAO analysis of FDA files.

Note: The sampling errors of the estimated percentages of 510(k) submissions reaching SE or NSE in FDA's decision-making process are within plus or minus 1 percentage point at the 95 percent confidence level.

[a] Performance data may be contained in the 510(k) submission, other 510(k) submissions, the center's classification files, or academic literature. In cases where FDA determines that performance data are not available, FDA requests data from the applicant.

[b] In 0.6 percent of the 5,063 cases, FDA made a determination of NSE, but the determination path is not represented in this flowchart. Reasons that these cases were found NSE include: the applicant failing to respond to an FDA data request and a PMA already being required for the device type.

Figure 9. Projected Percentages of 510(k) Submissions for Class II and Class III Devices in Fiscal Years 2005 through 2007 Reaching Each Point in FDA's Detailed Decision-Making Process

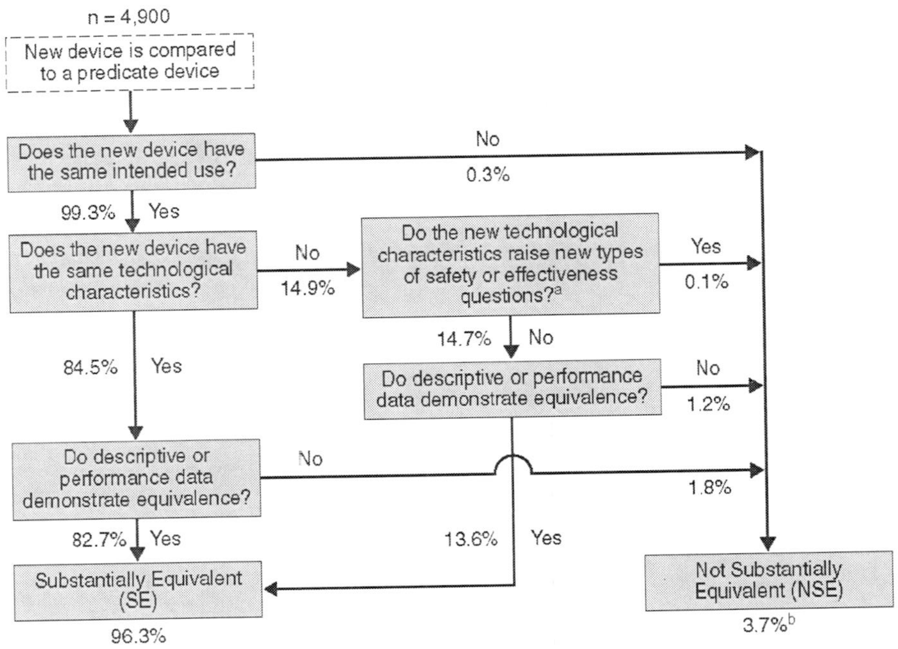

Source: GAO analysis of FDA files.

Notes: In cases where FDA determines that a new device has new technological characteristics that could not affect safety and effectiveness, the device may be determined SE if descriptive characteristics alone are precise enough to ensure equivalence. In cases where FDA determines that a new device has new technological characteristics that could affect safety and effectiveness, FDA requires performance data to demonstrate substantial equivalence. For cases in which descriptive or performance information is insufficient, FDA requests additional information.

The sampling errors of the estimated percentages of 510(k) submissions for class II devices reaching SE or NSE in FDA's decision-making process are within plus or minus 1 percentage point at the 95 percent confidence level.

[a] For devices with new technological characteristics, FDA first examines whether the new technological characteristics could affect safety or effectiveness.

[b] In 0.4 percent of the 4,900 class II cases, FDA made a determination of NSE, but the determination path is not represented in this flowchart. Reasons that these cases were found NSE include the applicant failing to respond to an FDA data request and a PMA already being required for the device type.

Figure 10. Projected Percentages of 510(k) Submissions for Class II Devices in Fiscal Years 2005 through 2007 Reaching Each Point in FDA's Decision-Making Process

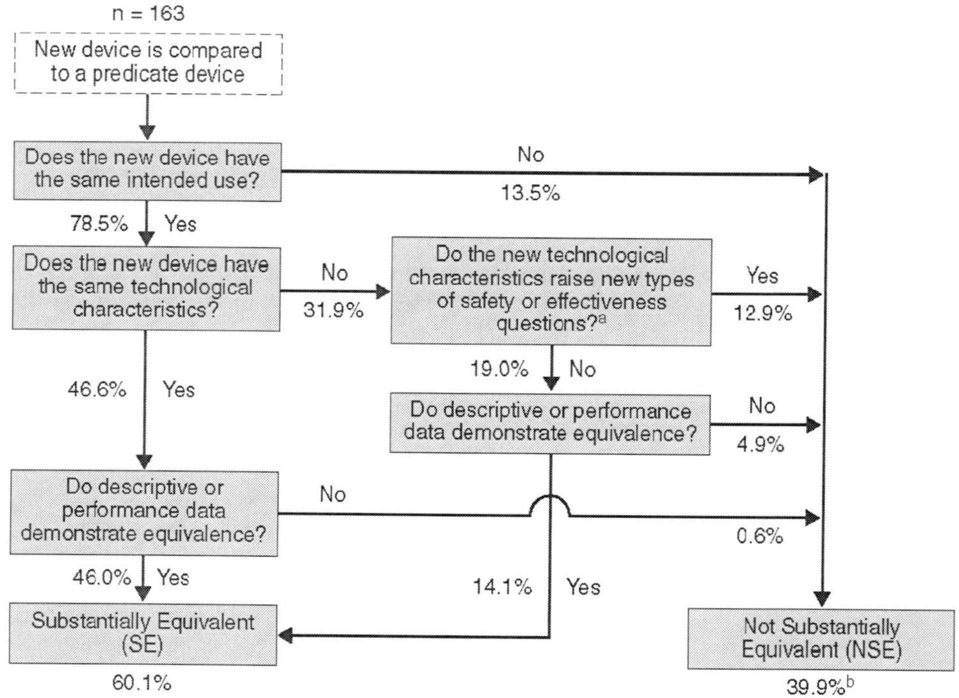

Source: GAO analysis of FDA files.

Notes: In cases where FDA determines that a new device has new technological characteristics that could not affect safety and effectiveness, the device may be determined SE if descriptive characteristics alone are precise enough to ensure equivalence. In cases where FDA determines that a new device has new technological characteristics that could affect safety and effectiveness, FDA requires performance data to demonstrate substantial equivalence. For cases in which descriptive or performance information is insufficient, FDA requests additional information.

Totals may not sum to 100 because of rounding.

[a] For devices with new technological characteristics, FDA first examines whether the new technological characteristics could affect safety or effectiveness.

[b] In 7.9 percent of the 163 class III cases, FDA made a determination of NSE, but the determination path is not represented in this flowchart. Reasons that these cases were found NSE include: the applicant failing to respond to an FDA data request and a PMA already being required for the device type.

Figure 11. Percentages of 510(k) Submissions for Class III Devices in Fiscal Years 2005 through 2007 Reaching Each Point in FDA's Decision-Making Process

Appendix VI. Comments from the Department of Health and Human Services

DEPARTMENT OF HEALTH & HUMAN SERVICES OFFICE OF THE SECRETARY

Assistant Secretary for Legislation
Washington, DC 20201

DEC 2 3 2008

Marcia Crosse
Director, Health Care
Government Accountability Office
441 G Street NW
Washington, DC 20548

Dear Ms. Crosse:

Enclosed are the Department's comments on the U.S. Government Accountability Office's (GAO) draft report entitled: "MEDICAL DEVICES: FDA Should Take Steps to Ensure That High-Risk Device Types Are Approved through the Most Stringent Premarket Review Process" (GAO-09-190).

The Department appreciates the opportunity to review and comment on this report before its publication.

Sincerely,

Jennifer R. Luong
for Vincent J. Ventimiglia, Jr.
Assistant Secretary for Legislation

Attachment

GENERAL COMMENTS OF THE U.S. DEPARTMENT OF HEALTH AND HUMAN SERVICES (HHS) ON THE U.S. GOVERNM,ENT ACCOUNTABILITY OFFICE'S (GAO) DRAFT REPORT ENTITLED: MEDICAL DEVICES: FDA SHOULD TAKE STEPS TO ENSURE THAT HIGH RISK DEVICE TYPES ARE APPROVED THROUGH THE MOST STRINGENT PREMARKET REVIEW PROCESS (GAO 09-190)

In general, we believe GAO's draft report fairly and accurately describes the Food and Drug Administration's (FDA) medical device premarket notification (510(k)) program. We agree with GAO's conclusions and recommendation to expeditiously take steps to either reclassify or call for PMAs for each class III device type currently allowed to enter the market through the premarket notification process.

FDA is committed to resolving the classification and premarket submission type for the remaining preamendment class III devices currently subject to 510(k). Since 1994, FDA has called for premarket approval applications (PMAs) or reclassified the majority of class III device types not requiring PMA at that time. In recent months, prior to the issuance of this report, FDA officials have met internally to discuss the most appropriate and expeditious method to require all class III device types to be approved through the PMA process. FDA is considering its legal and procedural options for completing this task as expeditiously as possible, consistent with available resources and competing priorities.

APPENDIX VII. GAO CONTACT AND STAFF ACKNOWLEDGMENTS

Acknowledgments

In addition to the contact named above, Kim Yamane, Assistant Director; Susannah Bloch; Matt Byer; Sean DeBlieck; Linda Galib; Julian Klazkin; and Dan Ries made key contributions to this report.

Related GAO Products

Medical Devices: FDA Faces Challenges in Conducting Inspections of Foreign Manufacturing Establishments. GAO-08-780T. Washington, D.C.: May 14, 2008.

Reprocessed Single-Use Medical Devices: FDA Oversight Has Increased, and Available Information Does Not Indicate That Use Presents an Elevated Health Risk. GAO-08-147. Washington, D.C.: January 31, 2008.

Medical Devices: Challenges for FDA in Conducting Manufacturer Inspections. GAO-08-428T. Washington, D.C.: January 29, 2008.

Medical Devices: FDA's Approval of Four Temporomandibular Joint Implants. GAO-07-996. Washington, D.C.: September 17, 2007.

Medical Devices: Status of FDA's Program for Inspections by Accredited Organizations. GAO-07-157. Washington, D.C.: January 5, 2007.

Food and Drug Administration: Limited Available Data Indicate That FDA Has Been Meeting Some Goals for Review of Medical Device Applications. GAO-05-1042. Washington, D.C.: September 30, 2005.
Food and Drug Administration: Data to Measure the Timeliness of Reviews of Medical Device Applications Are Limited. GAO-04-1022. Washington, D.C.: August 30, 2004.

GAO's Mission

The Government Accountability Office, the audit, evaluation, and investigative arm of Congress, exists to support Congress in meeting its constitutional responsibilities and to help improve the performance and accountability of the federal government for the American people. GAO examines the use of public funds; evaluates federal programs and policies; and provides analyses, recommendations, and other assistance to help Congress make informed oversight, policy, and funding decisions. GAO's commitment to good government is reflected in its core values of accountability, integrity, and reliability.

End Notes

[1] Generally, medical devices include items used for the diagnosis, cure, mitigation, treatment, or prevention of a disease. See 21 U.S.C. § 321(h). Throughout this report, the term *device* refers to a medical device that is not being regulated as a drug or a biological product.

[2] Throughout this report we refer to *type of device* or *device type* to indicate a generic category of device, which has a particular intended use (for example, a scalpel is intended to cut tissue) and which may include a variety of models made by different manufacturers. FDA's classifications of device types are codified in parts 862 through 892 of title 21 of the *Code of Federal Regulations*; in addition, FDA's Web site provides searchable databases. Class I devices are those for which compliance with general controls, such as good manufacturing practices specified in FDA's quality system regulation, are sufficient to provide reasonable assurance of their safety and effectiveness. Class II devices are subject to general controls and may also be subject to special controls, such as postmarket surveillance. Class II devices may support or sustain human life. For class II devices that are represented or purported to be used for those purposes, FDA must examine, identify, and describe the special controls necessary to provide assurance of their safety and effectiveness. Class III devices are those (1) for which insufficient information exists to determine whether general and special controls are sufficient to provide a reasonable assurance of the safety and effectiveness of the devices *and* (2) that support or sustain human life or are of substantial importance in preventing impairment of human health, or that present a potential unreasonable risk of illness or injury. See 21 U.S.C.§ 360c.

[3] A small percentage of devices enter the market by other means, such as through the humanitarian device exemption process that allows market entry, without adherence to certain requirements, for devices benefiting patients with rare diseases or conditions. See 21 U.S.C. § 360j(m), 21 C.F.R. pt. 814, subpart H (2008).

[4] *Substantial equivalence* or *substantially equivalent* means that the device has the same intended use as another legally marketed device and the same technological characteristics, or different technological characteristics and submitted information demonstrates that the device is as safe and effective as the legally marketed device and does not raise different questions of safety or effectiveness. See 21 U.S.C. § 360c(i)(1)(A).

[5] Some devices are exempt from premarket notification requirements. Most class I and some class II device types are in this exempt category. In these cases, the manufacturers must still register and list the devices with FDA.

[6] May 28, 1976, is the date of enactment of the Medical Device Amendments of 1976, which established the three device classes. See Pub. L. No. 94-295, 90 Stat. 539.

[7] Based on new information respecting a device, FDA may, upon its initiative or upon petition of an interested person, by regulation change the classification of a device from class III to (1) class II if it determines that special controls would provide reasonable assurance of the safety and effectiveness of the device and that general controls alone would not provide reasonable assurance of the safety and effectiveness of the device or (2) class I if FDA determines that general controls alone would provide reasonable assurance of the safety and effectiveness of the device. See 21 U.S.C. § 360c(e).

[8] Pub. L. No. 101-629, § 4(b), 104 Stat. 4511, 4515-17 (codified at 21 U.S.C. § 360c(i)).

[9] Pub. L. No. 110-85, § 225, 121 Stat. 823, 854.

[10] 21 U.S.C. § 360(k).

[11] Throughout this report, we refer to both submissions to FDA through the 5 10(k) process and applications to FDA through the PMA process as device submissions. Because related devices can be "bundled" together in a single submission, one submission may include one or more devices.

[12] The FDA-assigned product code for a device is based on the classification designated under the relevant classification regulations.

[13] For the purposes of this report, submissions for which FDA made *review decisions* include cases in which FDA made a determination to allow or disallow marketing of a device and cases in which FDA decided to discontinue consideration for other reasons such as if the manufacturer withdrew its submission. See app. I for additional information on our scope and methodology.

[14] Our analysis did not include certain types of device submissions, for example, special 5 10(k) submissions, which are requests for clearance of modifications to devices that have already been cleared through the 5 10(k) process. Panel-track PMA supplements are requests for approval for a significant change in design, performance, or use of a device, for which clinical data are generally necessary to provide a reasonable assurance of safety and effectiveness; 180-day PMA supplements are requests for approval for a significant change in components, materials, design, specification, software, color additive, or labeling.

[15] See app. I for additional information on our scope and methodology.

[16] See app. I for additional information on our scope and methodology. Some 510(k) submissions may be reviewed by third parties. For additional information on third-party review of 5 10(k) submissions, see app. II.

[17] Pub L. No. 94-295, § 2, 90 Stat. 539-41 (codified as amended at 21 U.S.C. § 360c(a)(1)).

[18] Before 1990, class II devices were defined as those for which general controls alone were insufficient to provide reasonable assurance of safety and effectiveness, but for which sufficient information existed for FDA to establish a "performance standard" to provide such assurance. Under the SMDA, this definition was revised to include those devices for which sufficient information existed for FDA to establish "special controls"—such as performance standards, postmarket surveillance, patient registries, guidelines, and FDA recommendations—to provide such assurance.

[19] Each manufacturer that wants to market a class I, II, or III device intended for human use for which premarket approval is not required must obtain marketing clearance by a 5 10(k) submission unless FDA issues a regulation stating that the device type is exempt from the 5 10(k) premarket notification requirements of the FDCA.

[20] Manufacturers are required to register with FDA within 30 days after operations begin and provide it with a list at that time of their devices intended for commercial distribution. Registrations and device listings must be updated annually. 21 U.S.C. § 360(j)(2)(A); 21 C.F.R. § 807.21 (2008).

[21] Regarding the devices listed with FDA that were not exempt from premarket review, about 31 percent (15,472) of the listed devices were allowed to enter the U.S. market through the 510(k) premarket notification process, and about 1 percent (529) of the listed devices were required to enter the U.S. market through the more stringent PMA process. Approximately 1 percent (389) were allowed to enter the market via other means, such as through the humanitarian device exemption process. A humanitarian device exemption requires a submission that is similar to a PMA submission, but does not include effectiveness requirements. FDA approval of a humanitarian device exemption authorizes the manufacturer to market a device intended to benefit patients in the treatment or diagnosis of a disease or condition that affects fewer than 4,000 individuals in the United States per year. See 21 U.S.C. § 360j(m); 21 C.F.R. pt. 814, subpart H.

[22] Pub. L. No. 94-295, 90 Stat. 539, 552-53 (codified at 21 U.S.C. § 360e).

[23] The act required FDA to promulgate regulations providing for the premarket approval of preamendment class III devices.

[24] For both preamendment and postamendment class III devices, after FDA issues a regulation setting an effective date requiring PMAs for a particular device type, all devices of that type must obtain an approved PMA to remain on the market. In addition, any new devices of the same type subsequently entering the market must also go through the PMA process—that is, they are no longer allowed to be cleared through the 510(k) process.

[25] After FDA reclassifies the device type into a lower class, the class I or class II device type would require clearance for the U.S. market through the 510(k) process unless FDA also exempted the device type from premarket notification requirements.

[26] For example, in 1988, GAO reported that FDA had called for premarket approval applications for only 9 of approximately 150 types of preamendment class III devices. See GAO, *Medical Devices: FDA's 510(k) Operations Could Be Improved*, GAO/PEMD-88-14 (Washington, D.C.: Aug. 17, 1988).

[27] The SMDA required that (1) FDA publish a proposed regulation regarding the classification of the device and provide reasonable opportunity for the submission of comments and (2) the final regulations regarding classification could not take effect until 90 days after the publication of a proposed regulation in the *Federal Register*.

[28] 21 U.S.C. § 360e(i)(3). The SMDA required the schedule to be established within 12 months of the effective date of the regulation requiring a device to remain in class III. Under the FDCA, in order to require PMAs for preamendment class III devices, FDA must take a number of steps, including publishing a notice of proposed rule making, allowing comments on the proposed rule, providing an opportunity to request reclassification of the device based on new information, and then publishing a final regulation requiring submission of PMAs. 21 U.S.C. § 360e(b).

[29] H.R. Rep. No. 10 1-808, at 6320 (1990).

[30] 59 *Fed. Reg*. 23731 (May 6, 1994).

[31] 21 C.F.R. § 807.92 (a)(3) (2008). Anyone submitting a 510(k) for a device type that has not been previously classified and which FDA subsequently classifies into class III, may, within 30 days after receiving notice of such classification, request that FDA reclassify the device under the statutory criteria for class I and class II devices. This process, known as the de novo classification process, permits FDA to establish a class I or II designation for devices that do not have a predicate and to allow them to enter the U.S. market and to serve as a predicate device for subsequent 510(k) submissions. 21 U.S.C. § 360c(f)(2).

[32] In addition to an FDA determination of SE or NSE, FDA may decide to discontinue its review for other reasons, for example, if the manufacturer withdraws its submission.

[33] According to FDA, performance testing should be submitted if there are important descriptive differences between the device and other devices of the same type or if the descriptive characteristics for the new device are not precise enough to ensure comparability. In these instances, the most appropriate bench testing, animal testing, or both to address the performance issue should be provided, and summary information regarding the testing should generally suffice.

[34] When clinical outcome can be reliably predicted from nonclinical data, well-designed bench testing or animal testing or both can be the basis for PMA approval.

[35] In addition to inspecting manufacturing establishments as part of its premarket review of original PMA submissions, FDA may also conduct inspections as part of the approval process for certain types of PMA supplements.

[36] For additional information on FDA's inspection of device manufacturing establishments, see GAO, *Medical Devices: Challenges for FDA in Conducting Manufacturer Inspections,* GAO-08-428T (Washington, D.C.: Jan. 29, 2008), and "Related GAO Products" at the end of this report.

[37] FDA's goals for original PMAs included panel-track PMA supplements. For 180-day PMA supplements, FDA's fiscal year 2009 goal is to review and decide upon 85 percent of submission within 180 days and 95 percent of them within 210 days.

[38] In fiscal year 2009, the standard fee for a panel-track supplement is $150,544 and the standard fee for a 180-day supplement is $30,109.

[39] See app. IV for additional information on 510(k) submissions for class III devices reviewed by FDA.

[40] See app. IV for additional information on 510(k) submissions for class III devices reviewed by FDA.

[41] For these device types, FDA determined that general controls alone were insufficient to provide reasonable assurance of safety and effectiveness and that sufficient information existed to establish special controls to provide such assurance.

[42] This includes two device types that FDA reclassified to class II under certain conditions, but retained the device type as class III that may be cleared through the 510(k) process for other conditions. For example, FDA reclassified endosseous dental implants to class II for root-form implants, but retained the blade-form implants as class III devices that may be cleared through the 510(k) process.

[43] All figures are estimates based on our sample of 510(k) submissions. Our analysis of FDA files did not include submissions for class I devices or submissions that did not receive a final determination, such as submissions that were withdrawn. See app. I for additional information on the scope of our review.

[44] In this report, we refer to both 510(k) submissions and PMA applications as *device submissions*. Because related devices can be "bundled" together in a single submission, one submission may include one or more devices.

[45] The FDA-assigned product code for a device is based on the relevant classification regulation.

[46] For the purposes of this report, *review decisions* include cases where FDA made a determination to allow or disallow marketing of a device and cases where FDA decided to discontinue consideration for other reasons.

[47] Our analysis also excluded de novo submissions. De novo submissions are for first-of-akind devices lacking a legally marketed predicate. Anyone submitting a 5 10(k) for a device type that has not been previously classified and which FDA subsequently classifies into class III may, within 30 days after receiving notice of such classification, request that FDA reclassify the device under the statutory criteria for class I and class II devices. The de novo classification process permits FDA to establish a class I or II designation for devices that do not have a predicate and allow them to enter the U.S. market. See 21 U.S.C. § 360c(f)(2).

[48] Pub. L. No. 105-115, § 210, 111 Stat. 2296, 2342 (1997).

[49] As of August 6, 2008, FDA listed 11 accredited third parties that can conduct third-party reviews of 5 10(k) submissions: (1) British Standards Institution; (2) Center for Measurement Standards of Industrial; (3) Cheiroon BV; (4) Citech; (5) Intertek Testing Services; (6) Kema Quality B.V.; (7) Niom-Scandanavian

Institute of Dental Materials; (8) Regulatory Technology Services, LLC; (9) TUV Rheinland of North America, Inc.; (10) TUV SUD America, Inc.; and (11) Underwriters Laboratories, Inc.

[50] FDA does not maintain data on the amount of these fees, which are negotiated between the 5 10(k) submitter and the third-party reviewer. However, FDA officials estimate the fee to generally be in the $5,000 to $10,000 range.

[51] FDA initially identified 154 device types that were eligible for third-party review. In March 2001, FDA expanded the program to allow third parties to review 5 10(k) submissions for many class II device types that were not previously eligible.

[52] 21 U.S.C. § 360m(a)(3)(A). In addition, in February 2001, FDA issued guidance stating that third parties may not review 510(k) submissions that require multiple FDA centers to review the device—for example, for drug-device combination products—or if a center other than the Center for Devices and Radiological Health, for example, the Center for Biologics Evaluation and Research, has the primary responsibility for the 510(k) review.

[53] FDA user fees for FDA review of medical device applications took effect at the beginning of fiscal year 2003.

[54] According to FDA, in fiscal year 2005 the difference in average review times between 5 10(k) submissions reviewed by third parties and 510(k) submissions reviewed entirely by FDA was 13 days, versus 45 days in fiscal year 2000.

[55] Before enactment of the SMDA, class II devices were defined as devices for which general controls alone were insufficient to provide reasonable assurance of safety and effectiveness, but for which sufficient information existed to establish a performance standard to provide such assurance. Under the SMDA, the definition was revised to include those devices for which sufficient information existed to establish special controls to provide such assurance. In addition to performance standards, special controls include postmarket surveillance, patient registries, guidelines and recommendations, and other appropriate actions as determined by FDA. The SMDA also stated that for class II devices that purported or represented to be used for supporting or sustaining human life, FDA was required to examine and identify the necessary special controls and describe how they would provide adequate assurance of safety and effectiveness.

[56] See app. IV for information on class III device types that were cleared through the 5 10(k) process in fiscal years 2003 through 2007.

Chapter 3

MEDICAL DEVICE USER FEES AND USER FEE ACTS*

Erin D. Williams

SUMMARY

The Food and Drug Administration (FDA) is the agency responsible for ensuring the safety and effectiveness of medical devices. An establishment may not market a device in the United States without FDA's prior approval or clearance.

In 2002, Congress first granted FDA the authority to collect user fees from medical device establishments. The authority was granted to help reduce the time required for the agency to review and make decisions about marketing applications. Lengthy review times harmed establishments, which waited to market devices, and patients, who waited to use them. User fee law provides a revenue stream for the agency, and also requires it to set *performance goals* for rapid application review.

The authority to collect medical device user fees has been authorized in five-year increments, and will expire next on October 1, 2012. In 2002, it was first established in the Medical Device User Fee and Modernization Act (MDUFMA; P.L. 107-250). Before reauthorization, it was amended by the Medical Device Technical Corrections Act (P.L. 108-214) and the Medical Device User Fee Stabilization Act of 2005 (P.L. 109-43). It has been reauthorized once, in the Medical Device User Fee Amendments of 2007 (MDUFA 2007), enacted as Title II of the Food and Drug Administration Amendments Act of 2007 (H.R. 3580; P.L. 110-85).

Since medical device user fees were first collected in FY2003, they have comprised an increasing proportion of FDA's device budget. In FY2003, $14.8 million of user fees comprised 6.8% of the budget. In FY2007 (the year of the most recent reauthorization), $35.2 million of user fees comprised 13.2% of the budget.

Medical device user fees have raised a number of issues. These have prompted Congress to determine the following: which activities should require fees; how user fees can be kept

---

* This is an edited, reformatted and augmented version of a CRS Report for Congress publication dated January 2009.

from supplanting federal funding, or being diverted from device review (through *triggers*); which activities the agency should fund with user fees; and how to qualify as a small business. (Small businesses pay reduced fee amounts.)

In addition to addressing the above issues, medical device user fee legislation has served a secondary purpose as a moving vehicle that legislators could use to address a range of issues related to medical devices. For example, MDUFA 2007 included provisions about the extent to which FDA can delegate activities to third parties (inspections and the review of premarket notifications); establishment registration requirements (timing and electronic submission); a unique device identification system; reporting requirements for devices linked to serious injuries or deaths; and requirements that FDA and GAO conduct certain studies. MDUFMA included provisions about reprocessed single use devices and other topics.

This report provides an overview of FDA and the medical device review process. It then presents the legislative history of user fees. Next, it explains the basics of FDA's medical device user fee system, noting the way in which various provisions have evolved. Finally, it provides an overview of non-user fee issues addressed in the device user fee acts. This report will be updated as events warrant.

Medical device user fees consist of congressionally authorized private money, which is paid by medical device establishments to the Food and Drug Administration (FDA). FDA is an agency within the Department of Health and Human Services (HHS). User fee funds are one of the two revenue streams available to FDA for carrying out its mission with respect to medical devices: to ensure devices' safety and effectiveness. The second revenue stream is direct appropriations from Congress.

Medical device establishments, to whom most regulations and fees apply, are often device manufacturers, but can also be domestic companies and importers who prepare and/or propagate devices. Establishments must obtain FDA approval or clearance before marketing their medical devices in the United States. They must continue to abide by FDA's requirements, including the payment of certain user fees, while their devices are on the market.

The authority to collect medical device user fees has been authorized in five-year increments. The same is true for the two other FDA user fee programs for prescription drugs and animal drugs.[1] The agency's authority to collect medical device user fees is set to expire on October 1, 2012.

Medical device user fees were first authorized in 2002. The Medical Device User Fee and Modernization Act (MDUFMA; P.L. 107-25 0) created the authorization. It inserted two new medical device user fee sections in the Federal Food, Drug and Cosmetic Act (FFDCA §§737- 738; 21 USC Chapter 9). MDUFMA was amended twice by smaller laws before its user fee authorities were reauthorized. These two laws were the Medical Device Technical Corrections Act (MDTCA; P.L. 108-2 14) and the Medical Device User Fee Stabilization Act of 2005 (MDUFSA; P.L. 109-43).

In 2007, MDUFMA's user fee authorities were reauthorized just before their expiration. The amendments came in the form of the Medical Device User Fee Amendments of 2007 (MDUFA 2007), enacted as Title II of the Food and Drug Administration Amendments Act of 2007 (FDAAA; H.R. 3580; P.L. 110-85).[2]

FDAAA was the most significant and sweeping piece of FDA legislation since the Food and Drug Administration Modernization Act (FDAMA; P.L. 105-115). FDAAA addressed topics ranging from food safety, to postmarket surveillance of drugs, to pediatric medical devices, to the formation of a nonprofit organization to assist FDA.

Two key factors converged to enable the passage of the broad legislation. The first was that significant FDA revenue streams would have been lost if its medical device and prescription drug user fees had not been reauthorized before their expiration at the end of FY2007. A failure to reauthorize the legislation would have cost the agency more than $280 million in user fees over five years. Reauthorization legislation was characterized as "must pass," providing a moving vehicle for Congress to address other concerns about FDA.

The second key factor leading to FDAAA was the emergence of a landscape of criticisms about the agency's response to safety concerns raised about a range of products the agency regulates. Publicized examples included adverse events related to products ranging from prescription drugs such as Vioxx, to medical devices such as cardiac stents, to imported items such as heparin and pet foods, to human foods such as spinach. Congress was able to address many of these threats to public safety in FDAAA.

Debates about which non-user fee topics were to be addressed in FDAAA and how they should be addressed slowed the process of reauthorization of FDA's authority to collect user fees. Those delays sparked concern that FDA would have to lay off some 2,000 employees due to the resulting funding shortfall, or at least issue legally required notices to the employees 60 days before such lay offs would have to occur.[3] However, neither layoffs nor notices were ultimately necessary. FDAAA was signed into law on September 27, 2007—four days before the user fee collection authorities would have expired.

Numerous topics of debate related to user fees have emerged over time. While many of these are related to the smaller details of the user fee program, three raise overarching policy issues for lawmakers. One concern is that the agency's reliance on funds collected from the establishments that it regulates could possibly create a conflict of interest. A second is that a reliance on fees could lead appropriators to give the agency less federal funding than they otherwise would.[4] A third is that the requirement that user fees only be expended on activities related to medical device approval drains resources needed for postmarket activities. Consideration of each of these issues will help to inform readers as they consider the details of the medical device user fee program described in this report.

The remainder of this report contains the following information. The first section presents background information about FDA's regulation of medical devices. The second section contains details about the medical device user fee acts and related key documents. The third section describes the way in which medical device user fees currently function, and provides relevant background for the various user fee provisions. The final section of the report discusses the various non-user fee topics that have been introduced or addressed in medical device user fee acts.

Background: FDA and Medical Device Regulation

In order to understand the function and impact of medical device user fees, and related policy issues, a basic understanding of the way that FDA reviews and regulates devices is useful. This section presents the definition of a medical device, an overview of the device industry, an introduction to the medical device components at FDA, and a survey of the agency's user-fee relevant requirements for medical device establishments, both before and after products come to market.

Medical Devices and the Device Industry

The first step to understanding FDA's regulation of medical devices is to see how the agency defines the term. According to statute, a medical device is

> an instrument, apparatus, implement, machine, contrivance, implant, in vitro reagent, or other similar or related article, including any component, part, or accessory, which is (1) recognized in the official National Formulary, or the United States Pharmacopeia, or any supplement to them, (2) intended for use in the diagnosis of disease or other conditions, or in the cure, mitigation, treatment, or prevention of disease, in man or other animals, or (3) intended to affect the structure or any function of the body of man or other animals, and which does not achieve its primary intended purposes through chemical action within or on the body of man or other animals and which is not dependent upon being metabolized for the achievement of its primary intended purposes.[5]

According to this definition, a medical device can be anything from a tongue depressor to a home pregnancy test to a wheelchair to a pacemaker. Types of medical devices vary widely, as do their respective levels of complexity and risk. Therefore, device manufacturing requirements vary significantly as well.

In part due to the diversity of medical devices themselves, medical device establishments tend to have certain characteristics. These characteristics can be highlighted by comparing the device industry with the pharmaceutical industry. The device industry is more fragmented and smaller than the pharmaceutical industry, with estimated earnings of $274 billion in 2007 compared with the drug industry's estimated $712 billion.[6] It is also dominated by smaller companies. These characteristics are important in discussions of user fees, particularly with regard to the way that fee amounts impact individual companies, and the effect that fees have on the development and review of new medical devices.

FDA Device Regulatory Structure

A brief structural overview of FDA provides background for understanding the way that FDA regulates medical devices, and for understanding the activities that require user fees. FDA has five regulatory centers, each focused on a particular type of product. The center within FDA primarily responsible for ensuring the safety and effectiveness of medical devices is the Center for Devices and Radiological Health (CDRH). One other center, the Center for Biologics Evaluation and Research (CBER), regulates some devices—specifically those associated with blood collection and processing procedures, as well as with cellular therapies (e.g., stem cell treatments). Jurisdiction of the centers' medical device review is governed by the FDA Intercenter Agreement between CBER and CDRH (October 31, 1991).[7]

Approval or Clearance of Medical Devices

Different types of applications to FDA trigger different user fees. These application types are highlighted in the following description of the way in which FDA classifies devices, and the mechanisms establishments can use to apply to market their devices.

CDRH categorizes medical devices according to their risk into one of three classes: Class I, II, and III. (See **Table 1**) The risk a device poses, and the regulatory controls required, increases from Class I to Class III. The device classification regulation defines the regulatory requirements for a general device type in each class. Most Class I devices are exempt from Premarket Notification and require only registration with FDA before marketing; most Class II devices require Premarket Notification (a 510(k)[8]) before marketing; and most Class III devices require Premarket Approval (PMA). Device applications are reviewed by CBER under biological license applications (BLAs). Devices on the market under 510(k)s have been *cleared* by FDA, while those on the market under a PMA or BLA have been *approved* by FDA.

Of all device-related submissions, a PMA (or Panel Track Supplement, which is described below) is the most rigorous and time-consuming application process for manufacturers and review process for the FDA. A 510(k) is significantly less rigorous, and is much more common. Most PMAs and some 510(k)s require clinical trials,[9] which are conducted with FDA permission via an investigational device exemption (IDE) that allows a device to be used in a clinical trial to gather information on its safety and effectiveness. The majority of medical devices that come to market do so with 510(k) clearance rather than PMA approval. (See **Table 2**) Applications to FDA for PMAs, BLAs, and 5 10(k)s all require user fees.

Device user fees are also required with four types of submissions FDA may require to supplement a PMA when there are changes in safety and effectiveness data: Panel Track Supplements, 180- Day Supplements, Real Time Supplements, and 30-Day Notices. Panel Track Supplements are akin to second entire PMAs. They reflect new indications for use or significant changes in device design or performance, and require substantial clinical data. An artificial heart valve approved for use to replace the aortic valve, and proposed for use in the mitral valve, would require the submission of a Panel Track Supplement. 180-Day Supplements are submitted for significant changes to medical device components, materials, designs, specifications, software, labeling, or color additives. A proposed change in a blood glucose monitoring system from wired to wireless telemetry would require this type of submission. Real Time Supplements are submitted when there are minor changes to the design, software, sterilization or labeling of a device. A change in the storage temperature and expiration dating for an injectable gel would require this type of supplement. 30-Day Notices are submitted for modifications to manufacturing processes or methods, such as a change in the sterilization process.

One alternative to a PMA that FDA offers also requires a fee: the Product Development Protocol (PDP). A PDP is based on early consultation between the sponsor and the FDA, leading to a device development and testing plan acceptable to both parties. It aims to minimize the risk that the sponsor will unknowingly pursue—with the associated waste of capital and other resources— the development of a device that FDA will not approve.

Table 1. Medical Device Approval Basics

Device Classification	Examples	Safety/Effectiveness Controls	Required Submission
Class I	elastic bandages, examination gloves, and hand-held surgical instruments	General Controls[a]	• *Registration only* unless 510(k) specifically required
Class II	powered wheelchairs, infusion pumps, and surgical drapes	General Controls & Special Controls[b]	• *510(k) clearance* unless exempt • *IDE possible*
Class III	heart valves, silicone gel-filled breast implants, and implanted cerebella stimulators	General Controls & Premarket Approval	• *PMA approval* unless 510(k) • specifically permitted *IDE possible*

a General controls include five elements: (1) establishment registration (use FDA Form 2891) of companies which are required to register under 21 CFR 807.20, such as manufacturers, distributors, repackagers and relabelers, and foreign firms; (2) medical device listing (use FDA Form 2892) with FDA of devices to be marketed; (3) manufacturing devices in accordance with Good Manufacturing Practices (GMPs) specified in 21 CFR 820; (4) labeling devices in accordance with labeling regulations in 21 CFR 801 or 809; and (5) submission of a premarket notification 510(k) before marketing a device. (Most Class I devices are exempt from the premarket notification requirements).

b Special controls may include special labeling requirements, mandatory and voluntary performance standards, and postmarket surveillance.

Table 2. Premarket Approvals (PMAs), Panel-Track Supplements, and Premarket Notification (510(k)s), FY2003-FY2008 Cohorts

Fiscal Year	PMAs and Panel-Track Supplements	510(k)s[a]
FY2003	50	3,795
FY2004	48	3,383
FY2005	58	3,401
FY2006	56	3,491
FY2007	37	3,036
FY2008	10	1,821

Source: FDA Office of Legislation. Counts include both CDRH and CBER workloads received through March 31, 2008.

a The receipt cohort is defined to exclude 510(k)s that were closed for any reason other than a decision to clear or not to clear a product under the 510(k) (e.g., when FDA finds that a 510(k) was not required). For this reason, some 510(k)s currently awaiting a decision may ultimately be excluded from the cohort.

One additional type of submission also requires a fee. It is a 513(g) request for classification information, so named because of the section of the FFDCA that regulates it.

513(g)s enable requesters to obtain information from FDA regarding the regulatory status of their devices or products.

FDA Postmarket Activities

In addition to receiving FDA clearance or approval prior to marketing, device establishments must meet certain requirements once their products are on the market. Many notable examples of this do not have an associated fee. For example, FDA inspects establishments where medical devices that are marketed in the United States are manufactured. Inspections assess compliance with FDA's *quality system requirements* for ensuring *good manufacturing practices* and other applicable specifications.[10] FDA also collects information about adverse events related to medical devices, and may request or require recalls of medical devices in certain circumstances. While no fee is associated with these functions, they are important to consumer protection, because they reflect the agency's efforts to help ensure that devices on the market meet required safety and effectiveness standards. In addition, they help to inform user-fee related policy discussions; the effect that user fees have on the agency's ability to conduct postmarket activities has been debated.

Two postmarket activities required of medical device establishments do have user fees associated with them. One is that establishments must register annually with FDA (*establishment registration*). The other is that establishments of certain class III devices must file periodic reports required by a PMA approval order (*periodic reporting*).

MEDICAL DEVICE USER FEE ACTS

Congress first authorized FDA to collect user fees from medical device manufacturers with the passage of MDUFMA in 2002. This was 20 years after a parallel authority had been granted for prescription drugs. As had been the case for drugs, the impetus behind authorizing user fees for medical devices was reducing the amount of time it took for FDA to make decisions about manufacturers' applications to market their products. The agency attributed the long review times to a shortage of funds to employ enough staff. The time taken in review affected patients, who waited for new products, and manufacturers, which waited to market the products. Manufacturers thus agreed to pay user fees (and Congress granted FDA the authority to collect them) so that FDA could hire more staff and decrease its review times. This section provides a historical overview of the laws Congress has passed related to medical device user fees: MDUFMA, MDTCA, MDUFSA, and MDUFA 2007. It also introduces two important related documents, the FDA Agreement and the Commitment Letter.

MDUFMA

In the years prior to MDUFMA's 2002 enactment, FDA's resources for its devices and radiological health program had increased at a lower rate than its costs.[11] As stated in the House Report to H.R. 3580 (MDUFMA):

> The medical device industry is growing rapidly. The complexity of medical device technology is increasing at an equally rapid pace. Unfortunately, FDA's device review program lacks the resources to keep up with the rapidly growing industry and changing technology. Because prompt approval and clearance of safe and effective medical devices is critical to improving public health, it is the sense of the Committee that adequate funding for the program is essential.[12]

In addition to issues raised by medical device review funding capabilities at FDA, prior to MDUFMA, concerns had also emerged regarding the reprocessing and re-use of medical devices that FDA had cleared or approved as *single use devices* (SUDs). Reprocessing means cleaning and sterilizing a device and verifying that it functions properly. Concerns about SUDs, funding, and the agency's capacity to inspect device establishments as frequently as required by law paved the way for congressional action in 2002.

In preparation for the enactment of MDUFMA, FDA officials met with industry leaders to agree upon mutually acceptable fee types, amounts, exceptions, and performance goals.[13] The agreement specified that, in return for the additional resources provided by medical device user fees, FDA was expected to meet performance goals defined in a November 14, 2002, letter from the HHS Secretary to the Chairmen and Ranking Minority Members of the Committee on Health, Education, Labor and Pensions of the U.S. Senate and the Committee on Energy and Commerce of the U.S. House of Representatives.[14]

MDUFMA was enacted in order to provide FDA "with the resources necessary to better review medical devices, to enact needed regulatory reforms so that medical device manufacturers can bring their safe and effective devices to the American people at an earlier time, and to ensure that reprocessed medical devices are as safe and effective as original devices."[15] MDUFMA amended the FFDCA to enact three significant provisions for medical devices: (1) it established user fees for premarket reviews of devices, (2) it allowed establishment inspections to be conducted by accredited persons (third parties), and (3) it instituted new regulatory requirements for reprocessed single-use devices.

KEY MDUFMA PROVISIONS:

device user fees authorized through FY2007
establishment inspections by third parties allowed
reprocessed single-use devices regulated

MDUFMA enabled FDA to collect over $133 million from medical device companies during the first five years of the program (FY2003-FY2007).

MDTCA

Prior to MDUFA 2007, MDUFMA was amended by two laws. The first of these was the Medical Device Technical Corrections Act (MDTCA, P.L. 108-214). It addressed three areas of MDUFMA.[16] First, it removed certain barriers to the third-party inspection program. Second, it amended an electronic labeling provision to extend the circumstances in which electronic labeling could be used. Third, it delayed the implementation of a provision that required a device to "prominently and conspicuously" bear the name of its manufacturer.

MDUFSA

The second law that amended MDUFMA prior to its reauthorization was the Medical Device User Fee Stabilization Act of 2005 (MDUFSA, P.L. 109-43). It contained five primary measures. First, it lowered *trigger* amounts of direct appropriations required for the agency to be able to collect user fees. Triggers are discussed in more detail below. Second, it changed the method of setting user fee amounts, eliminating the inflation, workload, compensating, and final year adjustments of revenues used for setting fees. Third, it allowed the HHS Secretary to use unobligated carryover balances from fees collected in previous fiscal years. Fourth, it made it easier for companies to qualify as small businesses and pay reduced user fees. Fifth, it deemed as misbranded (and thus subject to FFDCA penalties) any reprocessed SUD that did not identify the manufacturer, but allowed such information to be provided by a detachable label intended to be affixed to the medical record of a patient.

FDA Agreement

In preparation for MDUFA 2007, FDA and industry representatives met, as they had prior to MDUFMA, and discussed many of the above factors. They negotiated an agreement that they submitted to Congress ("FDA Agreement").[17] The Agreement contained legislative proposals as well as arguments to support those proposals. Pursuant to MDUFMA (§105), on April 30, 2007, FDA held a public meeting about the FDA Agreement. Attendees expressed general satisfaction with its terms. Congress incorporated most of the recommendations into MDUFA 2007.

MDUFA 2007

Congress addressed many issues in MDUFA 2007. Subtitle A reauthorized and amended FDA's authority to collect medical device related user fees. Subtitle B amended certain aspects of medical device regulation.

The primary issue addressed in MDUFA 2007 was the reauthorization of FDA's authority to collect user fees from medical device manufacturers. FDA's authority to collect these fees would have expired on October 1, 2007, if Congress had not acted. MDUFA 2007 extended the authority through October 1, 2012. The pending expiration of this authority was one of the primary drivers of MDUFA 2007 and FDAAA.

MDUFA addressed several other issues as well. One was to generate an increased and more stable user fee revenue stream for the agency with the addition of two new types of fees. MDUFMA had only authorized FDA to collect various *application fees*, which were payable upon submission of an application of FDA. According to FDA, there were fluctuations in the number of applications submitted from year to year, and fee revenues repeatedly fell short of expectations.[18] In order to address this issue, MDUFA 2007 added *establishment fees* (paid annually by each device establishment registered with FDA) and *product fees* (paid annually for each class III device for which periodic reporting was required pursuant to the PMA). MDUFA 2007 also added two new application fees and lowered the existing application fee amounts. The law was drafted to increase the total revenue generated by user fees, offsetting the lowered application fee amounts with revenue from the new fees.

KEY MDUFA 2007 PROVISIONS

device user fees authorized through FY2012
new fee types added
fee amounts reduced
qualification as a small business made easier

Another issue addressed by MDUFA 2007 was that domestic and foreign companies had expressed frustration with the difficulty in qualifying for small business user fee discounts. This led Congress to enact amendments designed to ease that process.

Commitment Letter

As was the case for MDUFMA, the requirements of MDUFA 2007 are supplemented by a "Commitment Letter" from the HHS Secretary, this one dated September 27, 2007.[19] The contents of the letter are incorporated into the law by reference.[20] The requirements of the law, as supplemented by the Commitment Letter, are summarized below.

MEDICAL DEVICE USER FEES

FDA has the authority to collect three types of medical device user fees:

application fees (paid each time an application is submitted),
establishment fees (paid annually by all non-exempt establishments), and
product fees (paid annually for each qualifying Class III device).

The authority to collect these fees will expire on October 1, 2012. This section presents the current law with respect to medical device user fees. Subsections describe the conditions under which FDA may collect user fees (triggers), how user fees relate to the medical device budget, which activities require and are exempt from fees, and the fee collection offset. They also describe the ways that fees may be used by FDA, fee-associated performance goals, required quarterly performance reports, the effect of fees on postmarket activities, and required annual reports to Congress.

Table 3. Medical Device Review Process Funding: Total Program Level and User Fee Funding, FY2003-FY2012 (dollars in thousands)

Fiscal Year	Total Program Level	Medical Device User Fees	User Fee/Total
FY2003 Actual	$217,285	$14,838	6.8%
FY2004 Actual	$179,245	$23,875	13.3%
FY2005 Actual	$244,282	$27,161	11.1%
FY2006 Actual	$255,041	$32,069	12.6%
FY2007 Actual	$267,543	$35,202	13.2%
FY2008 Enacted	$283,777	$48,431	17.1%
FY2009 Estimate	$290,921	$52,547	18.1%
FY2010 Authorized	not available	$57,014	—
FY2011 Authorized	not available	$61,860	—
FY2012 Authorized	not available	$67,118	—

Sources: FY 2003-FY2009: Food and Drug Administration tables for FY2005-FY2009, "ALL PURPOSE TABLE— Total Program Level"

This section presents current user fee law for each topic mentioned above. (For information on the history of each of the provisions in law, see **Appendix B**). Relevant citations to sections of MDUFA 2007 and MDUFMA are included parenthetically in the text, while those to the FFDCA and United States Code (USC) are included in footnotes.

Triggers

The authority to collect user fees is subject to two statutory triggers. If either trigger is not satisfied for a given fiscal year, FDA loses the authority to collect user fees. The first trigger places a requirement on Congress. It prohibits FDA from collecting fees if direct congressional appropriations to FDA for salaries and expenses related to devices and radiological health fall below a certain threshold. The trigger requires that, each fiscal year, FDA's salaries and expenses appropriation line for Devices and Radiological Health, exclusive of user fees, not be more than 1% below $205,720,000 multiplied by an inflation adjustment factor.[21] For FY2007, the year that user fees were last reauthorized, this translated into a minimum requirement of $229,334,000.[22]

The second trigger places a requirement on the HHS Secretary. It requires that fees only be collected and available to defray increases in the costs of the resources allocated for the process for the review of device applications. This requirement is considered to have been met each fiscal year if the costs funded by appropriations and allocated for the process for the review of device applications do not fall below specified levels.[23]

User Fees and the Device Review Budget

The amount of user fees collected has increased each year since collection was first authorized. MDUFMA fees comprised less than 7% of FDA's program level device review budget in FY2003, and over 13% in FY2007. The amounts are projected to continue to increase each year until the authorization expires in FY2012. In addition, almost every year since user fees were first introduced, they have constituted an increasing proportion of FDA's device-related budget. (See **Table 3**) Over the period of FY2003 to FY2007, the amount of user fees more than doubled, while the amount of direct appropriations increased by about a quarter. In FY2007, device user fees translated into 208 FTEs, or 15.6% of the FTEs in the device review process. (See **Table 4**) For FY2008, an increase of 37.6% in user fees is authorized above the FY2007 level. For each subsequent year through FY20 12, fee amounts are authorized to increase by 8.5% per year, generating a total of $287 million for FDA over five years.[24]

Activities Requiring Fees

Device establishments must pay fees when they submit certain types of applications to FDA for product clearance or approval, and must also pay two types of annual fees.[25] (See **Table 5**) The annual fees are an establishment registration fee (paid once each year by each manufacturer) and product fees (paid for each Class III device for which the PMA requires periodic reports to be filed). The annual fees are projected to generate about 50% of the total device fee revenue from FY2008-FY2012.[26]

The amount of each type of user fee, other than the establishment fee, is set as a percentage of the PMA fee,[27] also called the *base fee*. The law prescribes both the base fee amount for each fiscal year, and also the percentage of the base fee that constitutes most other fees. For example, a 30- day notice fee is equal to 1.6% of the base fee.

Table 4. Full Time Equivalents (FTEs) in the Medical Device Review Process, FY2003-FY2009

Fiscal Year	Total Device Review FTEs	Device User Fee/ Funded FTEs	Device User Fee Funded/ Total
FY2003 Actual	1,485	33	2.2%
FY2004 Actual	1,061	137	12.9%
FY2005 Actual	1,516	153	10.1%
FY2006 Actual	1,498	184	12.2%
FY2007 Actual	1,544	208	15.6%
FY2008 Enacted	1,546	208	15.5%
FY2009 Estimate	1,536	208	15.7%

Source: Food and Drug Administration tables for FY2005-FY2009, "ALL PURPOSE TABLE—Total Program Level"

As mentioned under the previous heading, the law raises the base fee (the PMA fee) annually by 8.5% per year from FY2008 to FY2012. (See **Table 5**) FDA asserts that this annual increase will ensure that fee revenues contribute their expected share to total program costs, and will provide industry with stability and predictability in the fee revenues it would expect to pay.[28] During the course of MDUFMA, from FY2003-FY2007, the rate of increase of the base fee (and thus the amounts of the contingent fees) slowed. It increased 34%

between FY2003 and FY2004, and 8% between FY2006 and FY2006. (See **Table B-1** in **Appendix B** for MDUFMA Base Fee Amounts.)

Table 5. MDUFMA/MDUFA 2007 Fee Schedule, FY2007-FY2012

Fees Structure	MDUFMA	MDUFA 2007				
	2007	2008	2009	2010	2011	2012
Application Fees						
PMA/BLA/PDP (i.e., *base fee*)	$281,600	$185,000	$200,725	$217,787	$236,298	$256,384
Small Business[a]	$107,008	$46,250	$50,181	$54,447	$59,075	$64,096
Panel Track Supplements	$281,600	$138,750	$150,544	$163,340	$177,224	$192,288
Small Business[a]	$107,008	$34,688	$37,636	$40,835	$44,306	$48,072
180-Day Supplements	$60,544	$27,750	$30,109	$32,668	$35,445	$38,458
Small Business[a]	$23,007	$6,938	$7,527	$8,167	$8,861	$9,614
Real Time Supplements	$20,275	$12,950	$14,051	$15,245	$16,541	$17,947
Small Business[a]	$7,705	$3,237	$3,512	$3,810	$4,134	$4,485
510(k)	$4,158	$3,404	$3,693	$4,007	$4,348	$4,717
Small Business[a]	$3,326	$1,702	$1,847	$2,004	$2,174	$2,359
30-Day Notice		$2,960	$3,212	$3,485	$3,781	$4,102
Small Business[a]		$1,480	$1,606	$1,742	$1,890	$2,051
513(g)		$2,498	$2,710	$2,940	$3,190	$3,461
Small Business[a]		$1,249	$1,355	$1,470	$1,595	$1,731
Product Fee						
Annual Fee for Periodic Report.		$6,475	$7,025	$7,623	$8,270	$8,973
Small Business[a]		$1,619	$1,756	$1,906	$2,068	$2,243
Establishment Fee						
Establishment		$1,706	$1,851	$2,008	$2,179	$2,364

Source: FDA, "Proposed Industry User Fee Schedule for MDUFA 2007," *Center for Devices and Radiological Health website*, updated April 16, 2007

[a] Small Business indicates the reduced small business fee associated with whatever item is listed above. (For more on the small business fee reduction, see the small business subsection below.)

Unlike the other fees, the amount of the establishment fee (also known as the *establishment registration fee*) is set in its own section of the law.[29] Like the other fees, it is authorized to rise 8.5% per year from FY2008-FY2012. (Earlier statistics do not exist, because the fee was first authorized for FY2008). In addition to the base fee increases, in one circumstance, the HHS Secretary has the authority to increase the fee amount of the newly created establishment fee up to an additional 8.5% (over the annual 8.5% increase) in FY2010. The HHS Secretary may do this if fewer than 12,250 establishments pay the fee in FY2009. This measure is designed to ensure that the fees collected from this source total 45% of total fee revenues, ensuring that FDA has a stable funding base from user fees.

Fee-Collection Offset

It is possible that in some years, the amount of fees collected will exceed the amount that FDA is authorized to collect. In that circumstance, for the four-year period of FY2008 through FY20 11, FDA may collect fees that exceed the authorized amount. A reduction is to be made in fees in FY20 12 only if the total amount collected in the four-year period exceeds the total amount authorized for the same period.[30] According to the FDA Agreement, this aggregation over four years will provide for greater financial stability for FDA than treating each year in isolation.

Fee Exceptions, Reductions, Refunds

Certain types of devices, sponsors, and manufacturers are exempt from certain fees, and small businesses pay a reduced rate.[31] These fee reductions, exemptions, and refunds are explained below.

Humanitarian Use Devices (HUDs)

HUD applications are exempt from user fees other than establishment fees.[32] An HUD is a device that is intended to treat or diagnose a disease or condition that affects fewer than 4,000 individuals in the United States per year. A device establishment's research and development costs could exceed its market returns for products to address diseases or conditions affecting small patient populations. HUD law provides an incentive for the development of devices for use in the treatment or diagnosis of diseases affecting these populations. A qualifying manufacturer may submit a humanitarian device exemption (HDE) application, which is similar in both form and content to a premarket approval (PMA) application, but is exempt from the effectiveness requirements of a PMA. Once on the market, certain follow-up measures related to effectiveness apply.

Devices Intended for Pediatric Use

In order to encourage the development of devices for use with children, any application for a device intended solely for pediatric use is exempt from fees other than establishment fees. If an applicant obtains an exemption under this provision, and later submits a supplement for adult use, that supplement is subject to the fee then in effect for an original PMA.

Applications from Federal or State Government Entities

Any application from a state or federal government entity is exempt from fees for a premarket application, premarket report, supplement, premarket notification submission, or establishment registration unless the device is to be distributed commercially. Indian tribes are exempted from having to pay establishment registration fees, unless the device is to be distributed commercially.

Further Manufacturing

In order to avoid the charging of multiple fees for a device that has multiple manufactured components, any application for a product licensed exclusively for further manufacturing use, is exempt from fees other than establishment fees.

Premarket Notification by Third Parties

Under authority created by FDAMA, FDA accredits third parties, authorizing them to conduct the primary review of 510(k)s for eligible devices.[33] The purpose of the program is to improve the efficiency and timeliness of FDA's 510(k) process, the process by which most medical devices receive marketing clearance in the United States. No FDA fee is assessed for premarket notification (510(k)) submissions reviewed by accredited third parties, although the third parties may themselves charge a fee for their services.

Small Businesses

Small businesses—those with gross receipts below a certain amount—pay reduced user fees and have some fees waived altogether.[34] These fee reductions and exemptions are important, because the majority of device establishments are small businesses.[35] According to the Government Accountability Office (GAO), the vast majority of companies that paid medical device user fees in 2006 qualified as small businesses:

> Of the 697 companies that qualified as small businesses under the MDUFMA user fee program in fiscal year 2006, 656, or about 95%, had revenues at or below $30 million—the threshold for small business qualification originally set by MDUFMA in 2002. Of the 41 companies that had revenues above $30 million but at or below the current threshold of $100 million, 35 had revenues above $30 million but at or below $70 million. Of the 697 companies that qualified as small businesses in fiscal year 2006, two-thirds submitted at least one device application subject to user fees during that year. These companies were responsible for about 20% of the approximately 4,500 device applications subject to user fees that were submitted to FDA in fiscal year 2006.[36]

An establishment is considered to be a small business if it has annual gross sales or receipts of $30 million or less. Proof of receipts may consist of IRS tax documents or qualifying documentation from a foreign government. Small businesses are exempt from fees for their first PMA, and pay at a rate of 25% of most other user fees, and 50% of premarket notification fees.[37] Small businesses must pay the full amount of the establishment fees. (See **Table 5**)

Modular PMA Refunds

Manufacturers may choose to submit to FDA the large amount of information required in a PMA in sections, over time, in a *modular PMA*. In the event that a manufacturer chooses to withdraw a modular application before FDA takes its first action on the application or before all of the parts have been submitted, the HHS Secretary may make a partial refund of the filing fee.[38]

Use of Fees

There are two different provisions that describe how FDA may use the device fees it collects. Both suggest that FDA may expend user fees on premarket approval activities, and not on postmarket surveillance. One provision was created by MDUFMA. It states that fees "shall only be collected and available to defray increases in the costs of the resources allocated for the *process for the review of device applications*."[39] The law specifies the elements of the "*process for the review of device applications*."[40] (See **Table 6**) They focus solely on activities involved in premarket approval. The one partial exception to this rule is the inclusion of the evaluation of postmarket studies that are required as a condition of approval.

MDUFA 2007 did not amend the above provision. However, §201(c) did include the statement in its findings that fees would "be dedicated toward expediting the process for the review of device applications *and for assuring the safety and effectiveness of devices*."[41] The law specifies that fees are to be used to support FDA in achieving the performance goals identified in the Commitment Letter. While it is conceivable that assuring the safety and effectiveness of devices could be interpreted to encompass postmarket surveillance, the Commitment Letter lists only premarket activities. MDUFMA (§101) contained similar specifications in its findings.

Table 6. The Process for the Review of Device Applications

The USC defines the process for the review of device applications as the following:
• premarket reviews;
• premarket inspections;
• monitoring of research relating to premarket reviews;
• review of *investigational new drug applications* (INDs) and *investigational device exemptions* (IDEs);
• monitoring of research conducted to develop INDs or IDEs;
• development of guidance, policy documents, and regulations to improve the process for the review of device applications;
• development of test methods and standards applicable to premarket reviews;
• technical assistance to applicants;
• initial classification or reclassification of a device;
• actions required to call for PMAs for Class III devices marketed before the Medical Device Amendments of 1976 (P.L. 94-295);
• evaluation of postmarket studies required as a condition of approval; and
• compiling, developing, and reviewing information concerning devices subject to premarket review to identify ffectiveness issues.

Source: 21 USC 379i(5); FFDCA 737(5).

Performance Goals

In addition to enabling the continued collection of user fees, user fee law requires FDA to meet new performance goals, which are articulated in the Commitment Letter.[42] These performance goals set general timetables for certain types of activities (such as PMA reviews), but allow for some flexibility that may be prudent, given that different types of PMAs and other applications may vary in complexity. Therefore, performance goals generally state that, for a certain percentage of applications, FDA will complete a particular type of activity within a given time period. (See **Table 7**)

Table 7. Comparison of Performance Goals in MDUFMA and MDUFA 2007

MDUFMA	MDUFA 2007
PMA and Panel Track Supplements	
50% of PMAs and panel track PMA supplements in 180 days	60% of PMAs and panel track PMA supplements in 180 days
90% of PMAs, panel track supplements, premarket reports in 320 days	90% of PMAs and panel track supplements in 295 days
N/A	50% of expedited PMAs and expedited panel track PMA supplements in 180 days
90% of expedited PMAs in 300 days	90% of expedited PMAs and expedited panel track PMA supplements in 280 days
Modular PMA	
N/A	75% of PMA modules in 90 days
N/A	90% of PMA modules in 120 days
510(k)s	
80% of 510(k)s in 90 days	90% of 510(k)s in 90 days
N/A	98% of 510(k)s in 150 days
180-Day PMA Supplements	
90% of 180-Day PMA supplements in 180 days	85% of 180-Day PMA supplements in 180 days 95% of 180-Day PMA supplements in 210 days
Real-Time PMA Supplements	
N/A	80% of Real-Time PMA Supplements in 60 days 90% of Real-Time PMA Supplements in 90 days
Biological License Applications	
90% of BLAs in 10 months 90% of BLA supplements in 10 months 90% of BLA resubmissions and BLA supplement resubmissions in two months	Same as MDUFMA

Source: FDA, "Comparison of Quantitative Decision Goals in MDUFMA I and II," CDRH website, updated April 16, 2007

In addition to the specific time-related goals presented in **Table 7**, the Commitment Letter also articulates several other goals. Four of these are related directly to the review process. One states that FDA will, at a minimum, maintain its current performance for processes for which quantitative goals were not identified (such as IDEs and 30-Day notices). Two others state that FDA will continue to incorporate an interactive review process for informal communication between FDA and sponsors to facilitate accurate and timely application reviews, and will make every effort to schedule both informal and formal meetings before and during the review process. In a fourth goal, the agency agrees to apply user fee revenue to support device reviewer training, as resources permit.

The Commitment Letter contains several other goals as well. Three relating to guidance documents state that FDA will update, or issue to the extent possible, guidance documents in accordance with the goals stated in the Commitment Letter, and will develop a guidance document regarding imaging devices with contrast agents or radiopharmaceuticals. In another, FDA agrees to facilitate the development of in vitro diagnostic devices (laboratory tests) by exploring ways to clarify the regulatory requirements and reduce the regulatory burden.

Performance Goal-Setting Process

FDA will be required to work with various stakeholders in order to develop performance goals and plans for meeting those goals in preparation for user fee reauthorization in 2012.[43] FDA will be required to consult with an array of governmental, professional, and consumer groups; publish its recommendations in the *Federal Register*; provide a public comment period; and hold a public meeting. In addition, the recommendations will have to be revised upon consideration of public comments, and transmitted to Congress not later than January 15, 2012.

Quarterly Performance Reports

The Commitment Letter states that FDA will report quarterly its progress toward meeting the quantitative performance goals. In addition, for all submission types, FDA will track total time (time with FDA plus time with the company) from receipt or filing to final decision (approval, denial, substantial equivalence [SE], or nonsubstantial equivalence [NSE]). FDA will also provide, on an annual basis, de-identified review performance data for the branch (section of reviewers grouped by subject-matter) with the shortest average review times and the branch with the longest average review times for 51 0(k)s, 1 80-day supplements, and real-time supplements.

Table 8. Appropriations Authorized for Postmarket Safety Information, FY2008-FY2012

FY2008	FY2009	FY2010	FY2011	FY2012
$7,100,000	$7,455,000	$7,827,750	$8,219,138	$8,630,094

Postmarket Safety

While FDA may not generally use medical device user fees to fund postmarket surveillance or safety activities, MDUFA 2007 (§212(h)) did separately authorize appropriations for postmarket safety information.[44] (See **Table 8**)

In preparation for MDUFA 2007, questions had been raised about the effect of MDUFMA on postmarket activities. According to FDA, MDUFMA focused on premarket review activities, largely limiting FDA's use of MDUFMA funds to this area, and focusing all performance goals on it as well.

Measuring the impact of user fees on enforcement activities is not a straightforward endeavor, and is beyond the scope of this report. For example, while one set of metrics (the number of CRDH warning letters issued each year since FY2000) shows that a decrease in the number of letters coincides with the start of MDUFMA, coincidence in time does not necessarily prove cause and effect. As is shown in Table 9, some of the recent decline in warning letters is due to a change in policy related to the Mammography Quality Standards Act (MQSA, P.L. 102-539).[45]

Annual Reports to Congress

MDUFA 2007 (§213) requires the Secretary to submit annual fiscal and performance reports for FY2008 through FY2012 to the Senate Committee on Health, Education, Labor and Pensions, and the House Committee on Energy and Commerce.[46]

Fiscal reports are to address the implementation of FDA's authority to collect medical device user fees, as well as FDA's use of the fees. Performance reports are to address FDA's progress toward and future plans for achieving the fee-related performance goals identified in the Commitment Letter. Performance reports are to include information on all previous cohorts for which the Secretary has not given a complete response on all device premarket applications, supplements, and premarket notifications in the cohort.

Non-User Fee Provisions Regarding the Regulation of Medical Devices Established in User Fee Acts

In addition to reauthorizing the collection of user fees, MDUFMA and MDUFA 2007 each amended various aspects of the regulation of medical devices. Some topics were addressed by both acts. Others were addressed only in one. This section provides information about the nonuser fee topics addressed in MDUFA 2007, and a listing of such topics addressed only in MDUFMA.

Non-user Fee Topics in MDUFA 2007

The non-user fee related topics in MDUFA 2007 were included in its Subtitle B. Some of these were also addressed in MDUFMA. Topics include third-party review of premarket notification, required registration and filings, a unique device identification system, reporting for devices linked to serious injuries or death, inspections by accredited persons, and several reports required from government agencies. The current state of the law with respect to each of these items is summarized below, highlighting the amendments made by MDUFA 2007.

Third-Party Review of Premarket Notification

Under the initial authority of FDAMA, the HHS Secretary has been authorized to accredit non- FDA employees to review applications for Class I and certain Class II devices.[47] This authority, as reauthorized in MDUFA 2007 (§221), is set to expire at the end of FY2012. According to FDA, the purpose of the accredited third-party (ATP) program is to improve the efficiency and timeliness of FDA's 510(k) process, the process by which most medical devices receive marketing clearance in the United States.

Under the program, persons may elect to submit a 510(k) to an ATP rather than directly to FDA. The ATP then conducts the primary review of the 510(k), and forwards its review, recommendation, and the 510(k) to FDA. By law, FDA must issue a final determination within 30 days after receiving the recommendation of an ATP. Submissions reviewed by ATPs are not subject to FDA user fees, though the ATP may charge its own fee. For 510(k)s submitted during FY2005, 510(k)s reviewed by Accredited Third Parties (ATPs) received FDA marketing clearance in an average of 81 days after initial receipt by the ATP—14% faster than comparable 510(k)s reviewed entirely by FDA (94 days).[48]

Required Registrations and Filings

In addition to registering annually with FDA, medical device establishments are required to provide the HHS Secretary a list of devices on which they perform specific functions (such as marketing or manufacturing).[49] MDUFA 2007 (§§222-223) restricts the list and establishment registration periods from October 1 to December 31 of each year, and reduces the list requirement from twice to once per year. MDUFA 2007 (§224) requires these registrations and listings to be submitted electronically, unless the HHS Secretary grants a waiver.[50]

Unique Device Identification System

The HHS Secretary is required by MDUFA 2007 (§226) to promulgate regulations establishing a unique identification system for medical devices.[51] The law contains no associated deadline. Such a system for medical devices might be used to help reduce medical errors, facilitate recalls, identify incompatibility with other devices or potential allergic reactions, improve inventory control, improve reimbursement, and reduce product counterfeiting.[52] Since 2004, FDA has required bar code labeling for drugs.

Table 9. CDRH Warning Letters Issued in Total and Under the MQSA, FY2000-FY2008

Fiscal Year	Non-MQSA	MQSA	Total
FY2000	191	337	528
FY2001	105	393	498
FY2002	75	206	285
FY2003	121	84	205
FY2004	193	5	198
FY2005	177	5	182
FY2006	149	5	154
FY2007	146	10	158
FY2008	164	2	166

Source: FDA Office of Legislation.

Prior to the passage of MDUFA 2007, the medical device identification encompassed four disparate elements.[53] One was the use of the universal product number (UPN), devised by the Department of Defense to streamline purchasing operations. A second was the use of a product data utility (PDU) to maintain accurate product data for electronic data interchange. A third was the use of auto-identification technologies, such as bar coding, that allow distributors and purchasers to electronically read UPNs or other identification information. And a fourth was the use of identification systems in some hospitals that can read UPNs and capture data or link UPNs to a PDU database. These types of medical device identification were quite disparate and had penetrated the market to widely varying degrees. Only a few hospitals were making use of identification systems in their operations.

Reporting for Devices Linked to Serious Injuries or Death

When MDUFA 2007 was passed, the law required the HHS Secretary to promulgate regulations requiring establishments to report to the Secretary if they became aware of information reasonably suggesting that their marketed device had or might have caused a serious injury or death.[54] MDUFA 2007 (§227) specifies the reporting requirements for such devices that have malfunctioned.

Accredited Third-Party Inspections

Accredited third-party inspections were introduced in MDUFMA (as amended by MDTCA) with the goal of reducing the burden on FDA inspectors by enabling FDA-accredited persons (third parties) to conduct certain inspections on FDA's behalf. Inspections play an important role at FDA. According to GAO:

> During quality system inspections, FDA investigators examine manufacturing controls, processes, and records. These inspections are FDA's primary means of assuring that the safety and effectiveness of medical devices are not jeopardized by poor manufacturing practices.[55]

MDUFA 2007 (§228) amended the accredited third-party inspection requirements, as described further below. According to the FDA Agreement, the amendments are aimed at increasing the quantity of useful information FDA has about the compliance status of medical devices marketed in the United States, and permitting FDA to focus its resources on inspecting those firms and products posing the greatest risk to public health.

FDA is required, by statute, to inspect certain domestic establishments where medical devices are manufactured at least once every two years.[56] According to a 2007 GAO report, FDA has not been meeting this requirement.[57] Instead, five or six years sometimes pass between FDA inspections at any one establishment.

FDA accredited the first third-party on March 11, 2004. As of May 31, 2008, 23 organizations had applied to conduct independent third-party inspections of establishments, of which 16 had received FDA accreditation. Since that time, 43 inspections of domestic establishments and one inspection of a foreign establishment have been conducted by accredited organizations jointly with FDA officials as part of training that FDA requires of accredited organizations. During this same period, 14 auditors from eight of these organizations completed the necessary training and were cleared to conduct independent inspections. As of May 31, 2008, these auditors had conducted 11 independent inspections—4 of domestic establishments and 7 of foreign establishments.[58]

GAO reports that several factors may influence manufacturers' interest in voluntarily requesting an inspection by an accredited organization:

> Potential incentives [to request inspection by an accredited organization] include the opportunity to reduce the number of inspections conducted to meet FDA and other countries' requirements and to control the scheduling of the inspection. Potential disincentives include bearing the cost for the inspection and uncertainty about the potential consequences of making a commitment to having an inspection to assess compliance with FDA requirements in the near future.[59]

MDUFA 2007 changed the third-party accredited person inspection program in three major ways. First, it streamlined administrative burdens associated with qualifying for the program. For example, for clearance to use a third party, the law now requires that firms provide FDA with 30 days prior notice of their intent to use a third party listed on FDA's website. Previously, a firm was required to petition FDA for such clearance.

Second, it made amendments designed to expand participation in the program. For example, the law now permits firms to use third parties for an unlimited number of consecutive inspections without seeking a waiver, with certain exceptions. Previously, the third-party program restricted qualified manufacturers of Class II and Class III medical devices to two consecutive third-party inspections, after which FDA was required to conduct the next inspection, unless the manufacturer petitioned and received a waiver from FDA.

The third change has to do with FDA's process for setting its inspection priorities. To do this, the agency uses a risk-based approach. To inform the risk-based approach, MDUFA 2007 requires FDA to accept certain reports that are voluntarily submitted by establishments. Establishments may submit reports by third parties that assess conformance with an appropriate international quality systems standard, such as those set by the International Standards Organization.[60] Previously, FDA did not accept such submissions.

Reports

MDUFA 2007 requires two reports by GAO and one by FDA to be delivered to Congress by September 27, 2008. One report is to present the results of a GAO study on the appropriate use of 510(k) clearance as a part of the device classification process to determine whether a new device is as safe and effective as a classified device. (§225) The second is to present the results of a GAO study on the number of *nosocomial infections* attributable to new and reused medical devices and the causes of such infections. (§229) MDUFA 2007 defines a nosocomial infection as an infection that is acquired while an individual is a patient at a hospital and was neither present nor incubating in the patient prior to receiving services in the hospital. The third report requires FDA to conduct consumer testing and determine whether labeling requirements for indoor tanning devices provide sufficient information to consumers regarding the risk of damage to eyes and skin. (§230)

Non-user Fee Topics Only in MDUFMA

The following issues were addressed in MDUFMA, but not in MDUFA 2007:

The review of combination products (products that combine elements of devices, drugs, or biologics) was to be coordinated by a new office in the Office of the Commissioner.

Electronic labeling was authorized for prescription devices intended to be used in health care facilities.

The sunset provision applicable to intended use based on labeling (§5 13(i)(1)(E)) was revoked.

MDUFMA explicitly provided for modular review of PMAs.

New provisions were added concerning devices intended for pediatric use.

GAO and the National Institutes of Health (NIH) were directed to prepare reports concerning breast implants.

The manufacturer of a device was required to be identified on the device

Appendix A. Acronyms Used in This Report

510(k)	Premarket Notification
513(g)	Request for Information About Device Classification
ADUFA	Animal Drug User Fee Act
BLA	Biological License Application
CBER	Center for Biologics Evaluation and Research
CDRH	Center for Devices and Radiological Health
CLIA	Clinical Laboratory Improvement Amendments (42 U.S.C. 263a)
FDA	United States Food and Drug Administration
FFDCA	Federal Food, Drug, and Cosmetic Act (21 U.S.C. Chapter 9)
FTE	Full Time Equivalent Employee
GAO	Government Accountability Office (formerly General Accounting Office)
GMP	Good Manufacturing Practice
HHS	United States Department of Health and Human Services
HUD	Humanitarian Use Device

IDE	Investigational Device Exemption
IND	Investigational New Drug Application
IVD	In Vitro Diagnostic Device (laboratory diagnostic test)
MDTCA	Medical Device Technical Corrections Act ()
MDUFMA	Medical Device User Fee and Modernization Act ()
MDUFA 2007	Medical Device User Fee Amendments of 2007 (, Title II).
MQSA	Mammography Quality Standards Act ()
MDUFSA	Medical Device User Fee Stabilization Act of 2005 ()
NSE	Non-Substantial Equivalence
OIVD	Office of In Vitro Diagnostic Device
PDP	Product Development Protocol
PDUFA	Prescription Drug User Fee Act
PL	Public Law
PMA	Premarket Approval
SE	Substantial Equivalence
SUD	Single-Use Device
USC	United States Code

Appendix B. History of MDUFA Provisions

This section contains a history of each of the user fee provisions. It presents topics in the same order and format used in the Medical Device User Fees section of this report, with one exception. The history of *Use of Fees* is presented in the main text with the explanation of the provision, not in this appendix, because the evolution of the provisions is relevant to their interpretation.

Triggers

The direct congressional appropriations trigger is lower than the one initially set in 2002. MDUFMA had required an appropriation equal to or greater than $205,720,000 multiplied by an inflation adjustment factor. (Current law requires 1% less than this amount). In 2005, legislation was required to enable the continuation of the MDUFMA user fee program because congressional appropriations had been lower than required for FY2003 and FY2004. MDUFSA (the 2005 legislation) lowered the MDUFMA triggers retroactively for FY2003 and FY2004, and prospectively for FY2005-FY2007, to the level required by current law. MDUFA 2007 perpetuated the MDUFSA trigger, including the adjustment factor, indefinitely.

The second trigger, for the HHS Secretary, was created by MDUFMA (§102) in 2002 and has not been amended.

User Fees and the Device Review Budget

MDUFMA (§102) first authorized the collection of fees in FY2003. MDUFA 2007 (§212(h)(1)) authorized an increase for each year between FY2007 and FY2012. The base fee amounts for FY2003-FY2007 are presented in **Table B-1**.

Activities Requiring Fees

All of the application fees except for the 30-Day Notice and 513(g) were authorized by MDUFMA (§102). As mentioned in the main text, in the lead up to MDUFA 2007, FDA claimed there had been fluctuations in the number of applications submitted from year to year, causing fee revenues to repeatedly fall short of expectations.[61] MDUFA 2007 (§212 (a)(1), (5)) authorized establishment and product fees, as well as two new types of application fees (for 30-Day Notices and 513(g)s) to help establish a more consistent and predictable user fee revenue stream for FDA.

MDUFA 2007 also changed the percentage of the base fee assigned to various types of activities, but the basic method of setting the fees is the same as it was under MDUFMA. The one exception to this is the way that the premarket notification fee (for 510(k) submissions) is set. Under MDUFMA, the premarket notification fee had been calculated annually, so that the total of all such fees, in aggregate, comprised a target amount. MDUFA 2007 provided that these fees are to be set like the others—as a percentage of the base fee.

MDUFA 2007 lowered the base fee by $96,600 in FY2008 from its FY2007 level. However, as noted previously, FDA projects that it will still have more fee revenue in FY2008 than FY2007 because the addition of revenue from the new types of fees should more than compensate for the money lost in fee reductions. The net effect should be an increase in fee revenue for FDA.

Fee-Collection Offset

The authority to consider excess funds in aggregate over several years was added by MDUFA 2007 (§212(h)(2)). Under MDUFMA, FDA was required to reduce fees in any year for which collections in the preceding year exceeded the amount authorized.

Fee Exceptions, Reductions, Refunds

The following is a history of the various device user fee exceptions, reductions and refunds.

Humanitarian Use Devices (HUDs)

MDUFMA (§102) created the HUD user fee exemption. MDUFA 2007 did not amend the HUD provisions. However, another FDAAA title, the Pediatric Medical Device Safety and Improvement Act of 2007 (Title III, §303), allowed that certain pediatric device manufacturers may also be able submit an HUD application.[62] The HUD fee waiver is not significant for manufacturers of pediatric medical devices. This is because under MDUFMA these manufacturers had already qualified for user fee exemptions as described in the next paragraph. The HUD fee waiver does not apply to the establishment registration fee created by MDUFA 2007 (§212(a)(5)).

Devices Intended for Pediatric Use

MDUFMA (§102) created the pediatric use exemption. It was not amended by MDUFA 2007, but the exemption does not apply to the new law's annual establishment fee (§212(a)(5)).

Table B-1. MDUFMA Base Fees (PMA), FY2003-FY2007

FY2003	FY2004	FY2005	FY2006	FY2007
$154,000	$206,811	$239,237	$259,600	$281,600

Source: "Fees" section, MDUFMA website of FDA's Center for Biologics Evaluation and Research, updated August 2, 2006

Applications from Federal or State Government Entities

This exemption was created by MDUFMA (§102). Unlike the other exemptions, MDUFA 2007 (§212(a)(5)) applied this one to establishment registration fees.

Further Manufacturing

MDUFMA (§102) created this exemption. MDUFA 2007 (§212(a)(5)) does not apply it to the newly created establishment registration fee.

Premarket Notification by Third Parties

MDUFMA (§102) created this exemption. MDUFA 2007 does not change the exemption, but Subtitle B (§221) extends third-party review authority from 2007 to 2012.

Small Businesses

MDUFMA (§102) authorized fee reductions for small businesses. MDUFA 2007 (§212(d), (e)) changed the details of the small business rules established under MDUFMA in two ways. First, it lowered the fee percentage that small businesses must pay. For example, as stated above, MDUFA 2007 requires a small business to pay 50% of the standard 510(k) fee and 25% of the standard PMA fee, whereas MDUFMA had required small businesses to pay 80% and 38%, respectively. (See **Table 5**)

Second, MDUFA 2007 made it easier for entities to qualify as small businesses with two amendments. The first removed MDUFMA's requirement that FDA consider the assets of partners and parent firms in the small business qualification calculation. The second broadened the types of acceptable gross receipt documentation beyond IRS filings, making it possible for foreign establishments to qualify as small businesses.

Modular PMA Refunds

This refund provision was added by MDUFA 2007 (§212(4)).

Performance Goals

MDUFMA (§102) and MDUFA 2007 (§212(g)) each incorporated the contents of a commitment letter into law by reference. According to the FDA Agreement, the MDUFA 2007 goals are fewer and more rigorous than those in MDUFMA. They build on the progress made in MDUFMA. In making these proposals, FDA considered efficiencies gained and expected by means of additional scientific, regulatory, and leadership training; additional staff, including those with expertise demanded by increasingly complex device reviews; expanded use of outside experts; and information technology improvements that allow FDA to better track and manage the device review process. Like MDUFA 2007, MDUFMA had created performance goals, which were articulated in the 2002 Commitment Letter. (See **Table 7**) According to the FDA Agreement, FDA was on track to meet nearly all of the MDUFMA performance goals, which expired on October 1, 2007.

Performance Goal-Setting Process

A performance goal-setting process was conducted in preparation for MDUFMA. A second one, required by MDUFMA (§105), was created in preparation for MDUFA 2007. MDUFA 2007 (§213) sets forth requirements for the third such process. The three processes and their requirements were similar, except that MDUFA 2007 added the requirements that the recommendations be revised upon consideration of public comments, and that the recommendations be transmitted to Congress not later than January 15, 2012. MDUFA 2007 also wrote all of the relevant consultation requirements into the FFDCA.

Quarterly Performance Reports

These reports were required according to the commitment letters issues pursuant to both MDUFMA and MDUFA 2007. Each letter specified a unique set of factors to be included in the reports.

Postmarket Safety

MDUFMA authorized additional appropriations for postmarket surveillance in the amounts of $3 million for FY2003, $6 million for FY2004, and "such sums as may be necessary" for FY2005 through FY2007. However, these sums were not appropriated. MDUFMA also required the HHS Secretary to conduct a study of the postmarket review impact of the medical device user-fee program. MDUFA 2007 changed both the amounts and wording of the purpose of the authorization for post-market safety appropriations.

Annual Reports to Congress

Annual reports were initially required by MDUFMA from the time that FDA was first granted the authority to collect medical device user fees through FY2007. However, MDUFA 2007 changed the law by requiring that the reports be made available to the public, by writing the report requirements into the FFDCA, and by expanding substantive requirements of the performance report.

End Notes

[1] See CRS Report RL33914, *The Prescription Drug User Fee Act (PDUFA): History, Reauthorization in 2007, and Effect on FDA, by Susan Thaul, and CRS Report RL34459, Animal Drug User Fee Programs*, by Sarah A. Lister.

[2] See CRS Report RL34465, *FDA Amendments Act of 2007 (P.L. 110-85)*, by Erin D. Williams and Susan Thaul.

[3] See "Prescription Drugs: FDA Could Issue Layoff Notices Without Prescription Drug User Fee Act Reauthorization," *Kaiser Daily Health Policy Report* (September 17, 2007)

[4] CRS Report RL34334, *The Food and Drug Administration: Budget and Statutory History, FY1980-FY2007*, coordinated by Judith A. Johnson.

[5] FFDCA 201(h); 21 U.S.C. 321(h).

[6] "Industry Profile," *Standard and Poor's Industry Survey Healthcare: Pharmaceuticals (April 24, 2008); "Industry Profile," Standard and Poor's Industry Survey on Healthcare: Products and Supplies* (March 13, 2008).

[7] FDA, "Devices Regulated by CBER" (updated March 15, 2007)

[8] 510(k), which is short hand for Premarket Notification, refers to the governing section of the FFDCA.

[9] For more information on the regulation and sharing of results from clinical trials, see CRS Report RL32832, *Clinical Trials Reporting and Publication, by Erin D. Williams, and CRS Report RL32909, Federal Protection for Human Research Subjects: An Analysis of the Common Rule and Its Interactions with FDA Regulations and the HIPAA Privacy Rule*, by Erin D. Williams.

[10] The regulations governing FDA's quality system requirements for ensuring good manufacturing practices can be found at 21 CFR 820.

[11] FDA, "Medical Device User Fee and Modernization Act; Public Meeting," *Federal Register*, vol. 72, no. 74, p. 19528, (April 18, 2007) at http://frwebgate6.access.gpo.gov/cgi-bin/PDFgate.cgi?WAISdocID=40432151607+2+1+0&WAISaction=retrieve, (hereinafter, "Public Meeting").

[12] U.S. Congress, "House Committee on Energy and Commerce, Medical Device User Fee and Modernization Act of 2002," H.Rept. 107-728, report to accompany H.R. 3580 , 107th Cong., 2nd sess., part 1 (Washington: GPO, 2002), p. 23.

[13] This process was similar to the one used previously during the enactment and reauthorization of the user fee act for prescription drugs, the Prescription Drug User Fee Act (PDUFA). For further information on PDUFA, see CRS Report RL33914, *The Prescription Drug User Fee Act (PDUFA): History, Reauthorization in 2007, and Effect on FDA*, by Susan Thaul.

[14] This letter is generally referred to as the 2002 "FDA Commitment Letter." See 148 Cong. Rec. H.R. 1(2002).

[15] Medical Device User Fee and Modernization Act of 2002, H.Rept. 107-728 (October 7, 2002), p. 21.

[16] For further information about MDTCA, see FDA, "Summary of the Medical Devices Technical Corrections Act (MDTCA)," (November 2004)

[17] Public Meeting.

[18] Public Meeting.

[19] "Commitment Letter" from Michael O. Leavitt to Edward M. Kennedy, September 27, 2007

[20] FDAAA §201(c).

[21] FFDCA 738(g); 21 USC 379j(g).

[22] FDA Office of Management, "Funding For MDUFMA and ADUFA Triggers," FY2007 Budget Formulation and Presentation, (February 22, 2006)

[23] FFDCA 738(h)(2)(B); 21 USC 379j(h)(2)(B).

[24] FFDCA 738(h)(3); 21 USC 379j(h)(3).

[25] FFDCA 738(a); 21 USC 279j(a).

[26] Public Meeting.

[27] A PMA is the most involved type of application that a device manufacturer could make to FDA (FFDCA § 738(a)(2)(A)). For more information, see CRS Report RL32826, *The Medical Device Approval Process and Related Legislative Issues*, by Erin D. Williams.

[28] Public Meeting.
[29] FFDCA 738(a)(3); 21 USC 379j(a)(3).
[30] FFDCA 738(h)(4); 21 USC 379j(h)(4).
[31] Unless otherwise noted with an alternate citation, all exceptions listed in this section can be found at FFDCA 738(a)(2)(B); 21 USC 379j(a)(2)(b).
[32] FFDCA 520(m); 21 USC 360j(m).
[33] FFDCA 523(c); 21 USC 360m(c).
[34] FFDCA 738(d),(e); 21 USC 379j(d),(e).
[35] Public Meeting.
[36] Government Accountability Office, "Food and Drug Administration: Revenue Information on Certain Companies Participating in the Medical Device User Fee Program," GAO-07-571R (March 30, 2007)
[37] FFCCA 738(d); 21 USC 379j(d).
[38] FFDCA 738(a)(2)(D); 21 USC 379j(a)(2)(D).
[39] Emphasis added. FFDCA 738(h)(2)(A)(ii); 21 USC 379j(h)(2)(A)(ii).
[40] Emphasis added. FFDCA 737(5); 21 USC 379i(5).
[41] Emphasis added. 21 USC 379i note.
[42] FFDCA 738(g); 21 USC 379j(g).
[43] FFDCA 738A(b); 21 USC 738A(b).
[44] FFDCA 738(h)(3); 21 USC 379j(h)(3).
[45] For more information about CDRH enforcement statistics, see the CDRH Charts in FDA Office of Enforcement, Office of Regulatory Affairs, "The Enforcement Story," (FY2006)
[46] FFDCA 738A; 21 USC 379j-1.
[47] FFDCA 523 (c); 21 USC 360m(c).
[48] FDA Office of Legislation. Numbers are the most recent available as of publication.
[49] FFDCA 510(b), (i)(1), (j)(2); 21 USC 360(b), (i)(1), (j)(2).
[50] FFDCA 510(p); 21 USC 360(p).
[51] FFDCA 519(f); 21 USC 360i(f).
[52] *ERG Final Report: Unique Identification for Medical Devices*, prepared for FDA by Eastern Research Group, Inc., March 22, 2006
[53] Id.
[54] FFDCA 519(a)(1); 21 USC 360i.
[55] Government Accountability Office, "Medical Devices: Status of FDA's Program for Inspections by Accredited Organizations," Report to Congress, GAO-07-157 (January 2007).
[56] FFDCA 510(h); 21USC 360(h).
[57] Government Accountability Office, "Medical Devices: Status of FDA's Program for Inspections by Accredited Organizations," Report to Congress, *GAO-07-157* (January 2007).
[58] FDA Office of Legislation.
[59] Government Accountability Office, "Medical Devices: Status of FDA's Program for Inspections by Accredited Organizations," Report to Congress, *GAO-07-157* (January 2007).
[60] The International Standards Organization (ISO) is the world's largest developer and publisher of international standards. ISO is a non-governmental organization that forms a bridge between the public and private sectors.

Chapter 4

THE MEDICAL DEVICE APPROVAL PROCESS AND RELATED LEGISLATIVE ISSUES*

Erin D. Williams

SUMMARY

The central medical device issue for Congress is how best to help speed medical devices to consumers if they are safe and effective, and correct them or keep them from consumers if they are not. A medical device may be anything from a tongue depressor to a pacemaker. In order to be legally marketed in the United States, medical devices must be approved by the Food and Drug Administration (FDA), the agency responsible for protecting the public health by assuring the safety, efficacy, and security of human medical devices and other products. FDA's Center for Devices and Radiological Health (CDRH) is primarily responsible for medical device review. The regulation of medical devices can affect their cost, quality, and availability in the health care system.

During reviews, FDA classifies devices according to the risk they pose to consumers. If a premarket review is warranted by the potential risk, a manufacturer must demonstrate that its device is safe and effective, or substantially equivalent to a device already on the market. FDA requires product manufacturers to register their facilities, list their devices with FDA, and follow general controls requirements. Manufacturers of FDA-approved devices are required to report serious adverse events associated with the use of their devices to FDA. In addition, tracking is required for some medical devices.

The medical device approval process is currently funded through direct FDA appropriations from Congress, and increasingly through user fees collected from applicants. FDA's authority to collect user fees, originally authorized in 2002 (P.L. 107-250), has been reauthorized in five-year increments. It will next expire on October 1, 2012, under the terms of the FDA Amendments Act of 2007 (P.L. 110-85).

---

* This is an edited, reformatted and augmented version of a CRS Report for Congress publication dated March 2009.

A number of medical device related topics are of interest to members of the 111th Congress. These include liability and preemption, the 501(k) clearance process, Medicare and other federal coverage, importation and inspection, advertising, the regulation of *in vitro* diagnostic products (IVDs, which are laboratory tests), and some other issues.

This report contains the legislative history of medical device regulation, describes FDA's approval process for medical devices, and provides an overview of the medical device related legislative issues facing Congress.

This report will be updated as events warrant.

INTRODUCTION

There are many dimensions to the central medical device issue confronting Congress: how to speed medical devices to consumers if they are safe and effective, and correct them or keep them from consumers if they are not. The goals of device availability and device safety may exert opposite pulls, with implications for consumers , the health care system, and the economy. Investment in medical device development reportedly reached a new high of $2.934 billion in 2006, and climbed dramatically again in 2007 to $4. 120 billion. However, investment slowed considerably in 2008, reaching only $2.85 billion during the first three quarters of the year.[1] The products generated by the nation's venture capital backed biotechnology and medical devices and equipment sectors supported nearly 494,000 high-skilled, high-wage jobs in 2006.[2]

Manufacturers make decisions about pursuing new devices based in part on the cost of their development. Additional regulatory requirements may escalate these costs, while other incentives, such as tax breaks or market exclusivity extensions, may diminish them. If the device development cost is too high, the eventual result may be that consumers are denied access because new products are not developed or brought to market. Access problems have led to proposals for and the enactment of incentives to develop medical devices for rare diseases and pediatric populations. However, if the regulation and oversight of device development are not stringent enough, unsafe or ineffective products may reach the market and cause harm to consumers.

Troubles related to medical devices can have serious consequences for consumers. Problems with the procedures and equipment for HIV (human immunodeficiency virus) and hepatitis C laboratory tests led to hundreds of incorrect test results in 2004.[3] Defects in other types of medical devices, such as pacemakers, defibrillators, and coronary stents, have caused patient deaths.[4] Consequences such as these have raised questions as to whether adequate enforcement tools, resources, and processes are in place to ensure that marketed devices are safe.

The federal agency primarily responsible for ensuring the safety and effectiveness of medical devices and certain other products (drugs and biologics, for example) is the Food and Drug Administration (FDA)—one agency within the Department of Health and Human Services (HHS). A manufacturer must receive FDA permission before its device can be legally marketed in the United States. FDA's Center for Devices and Radiological Health (CDRH) is primarily responsible for medical device review. One other center, the Center for Biologics Evaluation and Research (CBER), regulates some devices—specifically those associated with blood collection and processing procedures, as well as with cellular therapies (e.g., stem cell treatments). Jurisdiction of the centers' medical device review is governed by the FDA Intercenter Agreement between CBER and CDRH (October 31, 1991).[5]

FDA's medical device review process is funded through a combination of public money (direct FDA appropriations from Congress) and private money (*user fees* collected from device manufacturers), which together comprise FDA's device review budget program authority.[6]

Medical device user fees comprise a much greater share of the device budget now than they did when they were first collected in FY2003 (see **Table 1**).[7] Congress has reauthorized in five-year increments FDA's collection of medical device user fees. The authority and will next expire on October 1, 2012.

Medical device issues confronting the Congress arise in the context of a variety of concerns about FDA and CDRH.[8] Chief among these is that, in September of 2007, Congress passed the most comprehensive FDA reform legislation in almost a decade: the Food and Drug Administration Amendments Act of 2007 (FDAAA; P.L. 110-85).[9] The impact of FDAAA for medical device regulation is discussed below in the "History of Laws Governing Medical Device Regulation" section.

In the wake FDAAA, issues related to medical devices and other products remain both in areas that FDAAA did not comprehensively address, and in areas raised by its implementation. Most of these issues are discussed in this report. However, some FDA-wide issues, which are not discussed in detail, have consequences for medical device regulation. For example, questions have arisen as to whether FDA's budget is adequate for the agency to carry out its mission.[10] Reports have emerged of FDA scientists alleging that politics influenced medical device approvals, and that agency scientists' morale was declining.[11] In addition, in several well-publicized instances, FDA representatives failed to respond in a timely and candid manner to congressional inquiries.[12]

In order to fully understand the medical device related legislative issues that Congress faces, some background information is illustrative. This report provides an overview of the following: medical devices and their manufacturers, the history of FDAAA and other laws governing medical device regulation, and the medical device approval process. The final section surveys the device-related legislative issues of interest to Congress.

Table 1. Funding for the Device Review Process Salaries and Expenses, FY2003-FY2009

(dollars in thousands)			
	Total Program Level	**MDUFMA User Fees**	**MDUFMA /Total**
FY2003 Actual	$217,285	$14,838	6.8%
FY2004 Actual	$179,245	$23,875	13.3%
FY2005 Actual	$244,282	$27,161	11.1%
FY2006 Actual	$255,041	$32,069	12.6%
FY2007 Actual	$267,543	$36,861	13.8%
FY2008 Enacteda	$283,777	$45,785	16.1%
FY2009 Pres. Budget[a]	$290,921	$49,040	16.9%

Source: Food and Drug Administration tables for FY2005 - FY2009, "ALL PURPOSE TABLE - Total Program Level"

a. Numbers do not reflect the FY2008 Supplemental appropriation or the FY2009 CR.

MEDICAL DEVICES AND THEIR MANUFACTURERS

Medical device regulation is complex, in part because of the wide variety of items that are categorized as medical devices. They may be simple tools used during medical examinations, such as tongue depressors and thermometers. They may be high-tech life-saving implants like pacemakers and coronary stents. They may be machines used for diagnostic purposes, like CAT scans and EEG machines. They may even be test kits used in laboratories or by consumer at home, such as tests for pregnancy or blood glucose levels.

According to law, a medical device is an instrument, apparatus, implement, machine, contrivance, implant, in vitro reagent, or other similar or related article, including any component, part, or accessory, that (1) does not achieve its primary intended purposes through chemical action within or on the body of humans or other animals, (2) is not dependent upon being metabolized for the achievement of its primary intended purposes, and (3) is one of the following:

> recognized in the official National Formulary, or the United States Pharmacopeia, or any supplement to them;
> intended for use in the diagnosis of disease or other conditions, or in the cure, mitigation, treatment, or prevention of disease, in humans or other animals; or
> intended to affect the structure or any function of the body of man or other animals.[13]

The medical device market is highly fragmented: surgical and medical supplies make up the largest sector, followed by *in vitro* diagnostic products (IVDs, which are laboratory tests), cardiovascular devices, orthopedic devices, and diagnostic imaging.[14] Although the largest companies dominate the market for devices in terms of sales, it is often the small companies that make a significant contribution to early innovation. Small companies often partner with larger companies to bring products to market, because they often lack access to capital, and the resources to conduct clinical trials and navigate the regulatory and reimbursement hurdles.

These characteristics of the medical device industry distinguish it from the drug industry, which is less fragmented, larger, and dominated by larger companies. The U.S. medical device industry as a whole is much smaller than the U.S. pharmaceutical industry, with estimated earnings of $81.6 billion in 2007 compared to the drug industry's estimated $205.8 billion.[15] As a result, device companies often do not have the economic or financial resources of multi-billion dollar drug companies. These distinctions between device and drug manufacturers may be relevant in some regulatory discussions. Incentives and requirements placed on drug manufacturers are sometimes applied to device manufacturers as well, on which they may have a markedly different impact.

THE HISTORY OF LAWS GOVERNING MEDICAL DEVICE REGULATION

Though food has been regulated since early colonial times, and drugs since the Drug Importation Act of 1848, medical devices did not come under federal scrutiny until Congress passed the Federal Food, Drug and Cosmetic Act (FFDCA) of 1938 (P.L. 75-717). At that time, few medical devices existed. In 1966, the Fair Packaging and Labeling Act (P.L. 89-755) required all consumer products in interstate commerce to be labeled accurately and truthfully, with FDA enforcing the provisions on regulated medical products, including medical devices.

The Medical Device Amendments of 1976 (MDA; P.L. 94-295) was the first major legislation passed to ensure safety and effectiveness of medical devices, including diagnostic products, before they could be marketed. The amendments required manufacturers to register with FDA and follow quality control procedures in their manufacturing processes. Some products were required to undergo premarket review by FDA, while others had to meet performance standards before marketing. Devices already on the market in 1976 (*preamendment* or *grandfathered* devices) did not have to undergo retrospective approval for marketing. Instead, they were to be broadly classified by FDA into one of three regulatory classes based on the risk they posed to the patient. Devices coming to market after 1976 had to undergo premarket review (unless they were exempt). Devices could be *cleared* by FDA if they were substantially equivalent to a preamendment device. If the device (or its use) were truly novel, it could be *approved* if it was proven safe and effective on its own merits.

In 1990, the Safe Medical Devices Act (SMD Act; P.L. 101-629) established postmarket requirements for medical devices. The SMD Act required facilities that use medical devices to report to FDA any incident that suggested that a medical device could have caused or contributed to the death, serious illness, or injury of a patient. Manufacturers of certain permanently implanted devices were required to establish methods for tracking the patients who received them and to conduct postmarket surveillance to identify adverse events. The act authorized FDA to carry out certain enforcement actions, such as device product recalls, for products that did not comply with the law.

In 1997, the Food and Drug Administration Modernization Act (FDAMA; P.L. 105-115) mandated the most wide-ranging reforms in FDA practice since 1938. For medical devices, provisions included measures to accelerate premarket review of devices and to regulate company advertising of unapproved uses of approved devices.

In 2002, the Medical Device User Fee and Modernization Act (MDUFMA; P.L. 107-250) amended the FFDCA to enact three significant provisions for medical devices: (1) it established user fees for premarket reviews of devices; (2) it allowed establishment inspections to be conducted by accredited persons (third parties); and (3) it instituted new regulatory requirements for reprocessed single-use devices. MDUFMA was amended and clarified by two laws: the Medical Device Technical Corrections Act (MDTCA, P.L. 108-214), and the Medical Device User Fee Stabilization Act of 2005 (MDUFSA, P.L. 109-43), and had its user fee provisions reauthorized by FDAAA.[16]

In 2007, FDAAA amended the FFDCA and the Public Health Service Act to reauthorize several expiring programs (including the medical device user fee act) and to make agency-wide changes, several of which have implications for the regulation of medical devices.[17]

FDAAA created incentives as well as reporting and safety requirements for manufacturers of medical devices for children; required that certain clinical trials for medical devices and some other products be publicly registered and have their results posted;[18] created requirements to reduce conflicts of interest in advisory committees for medical devices and other products;[19] and made certain other amendments to the regulation of devices.

The Medical Device Approval Process: Premarket Review Requirements

In order for medical devices to be marketed in the United States, manufacturers[20] must register and list the devices that they commercialize with FDA, and for most devices, must obtain the agency's prior and continuing permission.[21] FDA grants this permission when a manufacturer meets regulatory premarket and postmarket requirements. The premarket requirements, which are the subject of this section, vary according to a the risk that a device presents. IVDs have their own unique premarket requirements.

FDA may grant a manufacturer permission to market a device after conducting a premarket review, based on an application from the manufacturer. There are numerous types of applications a manufacturer can submit to obtain such permission, which are described later in this section. First, however, this section presents some fundamental concepts and terms of art that will help readers to understand the details of the various application processes. These include *safety* and *effectiveness*, *approval* and *clearance* (including *substantial equivalence* to a *predicate device*), and device *classification* (including types of *controls*).

Fundamental Concepts and Terms of Art

Safety and Effectiveness

FDA has as a part of its mission to ensure that medical devices are *safe* and *effective*. The evidence required to meet the safe and effective standard varies according to the characteristics of the device, its conditions of use, the existence and adequacy of warnings and other restrictions, and the extent of experience with its use.[22] FDA considers there to be reasonable assurance of safety when it can be determined that the probable benefits to health that result from use of the device as directed by the manufacturer outweigh any probable risks.[23] Investigations for safety can include animal studies, human studies, and/or laboratory studies.[24]

FDA considers there to be reasonable assurance of effectiveness when valid scientific evidence suggests that the target population's use of the device (according to the manufacturer's instructions) provides clinically significant results.[25] Valid scientific evidence includes that from controlled clinical trials, other carefully defined clinical investigations, case histories, and other reports of significant human experience. Evidence can be collected by the manufacturer or a representative, and can be abstracted from medical literature.

Approval and Clearance

There are two paths that manufacturers can use to bring their medical devices to market with FDA's permission. One path consists of conducting clinical studies comparable to those required for new prescription drugs. This process, generally used for novel and high-risk devices, is typically lengthy and expensive. It results in a type of FDA permission called *approval.*

The other path is to demonstrate that the device is *substantially equivalent* to a device that is already on the market (a *predicate device*).[26] This type of process is unique to medical devices. It is typically used for new devices that make incremental improvements or modifications to previous versions. It results in FDA *clearance,* and tends to be much less expensive and less time- consuming than seeking FDA approval.

Substantial equivalence is determined by comparing the performance characteristics of a new device with those of a predicate device. To be considered substantially equivalent, FDA must determine that the new device has the same *intended use* (also called *indication(s) for use*) as a predicate device.[27] In addition, the new device must either (1) have the same technological characteristics as the predicate, (2) have different technological characteristics that do not raise new questions of safety and effectiveness, or (3) be least as safe and effective as the predicate. The manufacturer selects which predicate device to compare with its new device. However, FDA has the ultimate discretion in determining whether a comparison is appropriate.

Here is an example of how a device might be cleared through a determination of substantial equivalence. If a manufacturer wanted to market a blood glucose test for diabetes, it could apply to FDA for a determination that the new device is substantially equivalent to a blood glucose test for diabetes that was sold in 1972. FDA has classified these devices in the Code of Federal Regulations (CFR) as follows (note, the device classification process is described at the start of the next section):

> 21 CFR 862.1345 Glucose test system.
>
> (a) Identification. A glucose test system is a device intended to measure glucose quantitatively in blood and other body fluids. Glucose measurements are used in the diagnosis and treatment of carbohydrate metabolism disorders including diabetes mellitus, neonatal hypoglycemia, and idiopathic hypoglycemia, and of pancreatic islet cell carcinoma.
>
> (b) Classification. Class II.

The manufacturer would likely ask FDA to clear the new device based on evidence that it was substantially equivalent to the device described in the CFR, rather than based on a large-scale clinical study. To obtain FDA clearance, the manufacturer would need to demonstrate two things. First, that the new device did not present new questions of safety and effectiveness. Second, that it had the same intended use as the older device (i.e., "... intended to measure glucose quantitatively in blood and other body fluids.... "). If, based on the evidence, FDA determined that the new device was substantially equivalent to the predicate, the agency could clear the new device, and the manufacturer could market it.

Device Classification

Under the terms of the MDA, FDA has created three broad categories to describe the risk that each medical device poses to its intended patients (the *target population*) when it is used or misused.[28] The risk categories (known as *classifications*) are *Class I*, *II* , and *III*, which represent low-, moderate-, and high-risk categories, respectively. (See **Table 2**.) Since the MDA was enacted, the agency has classified over 1,700 distinct types of devices and organized them in the Code of Federal regulations (CFR) in 16 medical specialties (referred to as *classification panels*), such as "cardiovascular devices" or "ear, nose, and throat devices."

FDA can classify a new device based on comparison with a legally marketed device, by regulation, or by recognizing that if falls into a classification panel. If unsure what classification a product would receive, a manufacturer may make a formal request for classification to FDA.

A device's classification determines the type of regulatory requirements that a manufacturer must follow.[29] These regulatory requirements, known as *controls*, are described in more in the descriptions of Class I, II, and II devices that follows.

Class I

Devices in Class I are those for which *general controls* are sufficient to ensure their safe and effective use (21 CFR § 860.3(c)(1)). General controls, the minimum regulations that apply to all FDA regulated medical devices, include five elements:[30]

> *establishment registration*—registration with FDA of companies required to do so under 21 CFR 807.20 (such as manufacturers, distributors, repackagers and relabelers, and foreign firms);
>
> *device listing*—listing with FDA of all devices to be marketed;
>
> good manufacturing practices (GMP)—manufacturing of devices in accordance with the Quality Systems Regulation (QSR) in 21 CFR 820;
>
> *labeling*—labeling of devices in accordance with 21 CFR 801 or 809; and
>
> *premarket notification*—submission to FDA of a premarket notification 510(k) (described in detail in the *Types of Device Marketing Applications* section below).

Many Class I devices are *exempt* from the premarket notification and/or the QSR requirements, though they still have to comply with the other general controls. A device is exempt if FDA determines that it presents a low risk of illness or injury to patients. (See 21 CFR 862 to 892).

Class II

Devices in Class II are those for which general controls alone are not sufficient to provide reasonable assurance of safety and effectiveness. Class II includes devices that pose a moderate risk to patients, and may include new devices for which information or *special controls* are available to reduce or mitigate risk. Most Class II devices require premarket review; however, some are exempt by regulation (21 CFR 860.3(c)(2)).

Special controls are requirements beyond general controls that FDA deems necessary to assure safe and effective use of a medical device (FFDCA 513(a)(1)(B)). They might include, for example, performance standards, postmarket surveillance requirements, or patient registries, or the development and dissemination of guidelines.

Class III

Class III medical devices include those for which general and/or special controls are not sufficient to assure safe and effective use of the device, and which require *premarket approval* (described in detail in the *Medical Device Marketing Applications* section below; FFDCA 51 3(a)(1)(C)). Class III includes devices which are life-supporting or life-sustaining, and devices which present a high or potentially unreasonable risk of illness or injury to a patient. New devices that are not classified as Class I or II by another means, are automatically designated as Class III unless the manufacturer files a request or petition for reclassification under FFDCA 513(f)(2). (Also see 21 CFR 860.3(c)(3)).

Medical Device Marketing Applications

As stated above, a manufacturer can market a device if FDA determines that the device is safe and effective. The agency makes that determination based on information the manufacturer submits. The information that is required—in other words, the type of marketing application the manufacturer must make (if any)—is determined based on the *risk* of that the device poses, if used according to the manufacturer's instructions. Under the terms of MDUFMA and FDAAA, manufacturers must pay a fee for most types of submissions.[31]

Generally speaking, according to the FFDCA, manufacturers:

are prohibited from selling an adulterated product;[32]
are prohibited from misbranding a product;[33]
must register their facility with FDA and list all of the medical devices that they produce or process (a process which now requires a fee under the terms of FDAAA);
must file the appropriate premarket submission with the agency at least 90 days before introducing a *non-exempt* device onto the market; and
must report to FDA any incident that they are aware of that suggests that their device may have caused or contributed to a death or serious injury.

Very few applications are actually denied approval. Instead, an application may be deemed "not approvable" in its current form (typically because the data that the manufacturer provides are not sufficient to demonstrate safety and effectiveness). Applications that are "not approvable" are usually withdrawn by the manufacturer before a denial is rendered.

Table 2. Medical Device Approval Basics

Device Classification	Examples	Safety / Effectiveness Controls	Required Submission[a]
Class I	elastic bandages, examination gloves, and hand-held surgical instruments	General Controls	• *Registration only* unless 510(k) specifically required
Class II	powered wheelchairs, infusion pumps, and surgical drapes	General Controls & Special Controls[b]	• *510(k) clearance* unless exempt • *IDE* possible
Class III	heart valves, silicone gel-filled breast implants, and implanted cerebella stimulators	General Controls & Premarket Approval	• *PMA approval* unless 510(k) specifically permitted • *IDE probable*

a. Each type of required submissions is described in the *Types of Device Marketing Applications* section that follows.

b. Special controls are described in the Class II section below.

Before a Marketing Application Is Submitted

FDAMA gave FDA the authority to establish procedures for meeting with manufacturers prior to preparing a submission.[34] The procedures aim to speed the review process by giving FDA and a manufacturer the opportunity to address questions and concerns about the device and/or the planned studies that will be used to support the marketing application before the studies are initiated and the application is submitted. For example, the "pre-IDE" process (an IDE is an investigational device exemption that allows a manufacturer to conduct a clinical trial on a medical device) is an informal "pre-submission" process. The "pre-IDE" process is so-called in name only; submitting a pre-IDE does not mean that manufacturers are required to submit subsequently an IDE application.[35] The pre-IDE process is simply a means for FDA and industry to engage in dialogue about a new device, before a study is initiated or a marketing application is submitted.

The pre-IDE process may involve sending analytical or clinical protocols to FDA for review and comment before proceeding with studies, or meeting with FDA to discuss protocols and/or possible regulatory pathways. This particular process is strictly voluntary, and not binding on either FDA or industry. The benefits to manufacturers include an opportunity to begin a dialogue with FDA, to promote greater understanding of new technologies, to reduce the cost of research studies by focusing on the important information needed for FDA approval (or clearance), eliminating unnecessary or burdensome studies, and to speed the review process for the future marketing application since FDA will already be familiar with the device.

Marketing Applications for Medical Devices

The following sections describe the types of premarket submissions that FDA reviews for medical devices. (See **Table 2**).

Premarket Notification (510(k))

A 510(k) submission is required for any new, non-exempt low- or moderate-risk medical device that will be marketed in the United States. A 510(k) could also be used for currently marketed devices for which the manufacturer seeks a new indication (e.g., a new population, such as pediatric use, or a new disease or condition), or for which the manufacturer has changed the design or technical characteristics such that the change may affect the performance characteristics of the device.

The standard for clearance of a traditional 510(k) is substantial equivalence with a predicate device. A predicate device can be one of two things. It can be a previously cleared Class I or II device that does not require a PMA. It can also be preamendment Class III for which the agency has not issued regulations requiring a PMA. (PMAs, which are more rigorous submissions than 510(k)s, are discussed in the next section.)

There are several types of 510(k)s: traditional, abbreviated, special and *de novo*. In a traditional 510(k), the manufacturer submits information about the performance of the device under specific conditions of use. It also contains information about the design of the device, characteristics of device components, representations of packaging and labeling, a description and summary of the non-clinical and clinical studies that were done to support the device performance characteristics, a description of means by which users can assess the quality of the device, and information about any computer software or additional or special equipment needed. Several administrative forms are also required.[36]

Most of the studies supporting a 510(k) submission are not true clinical studies. While FDA prefers to see data on performance of the device in the actual intended population, substantial equivalence in many cases, means only that the device performs in a similar fashion to the predicate under a similar set of circumstances. As a result, many devices never have to demonstrate safety and effectiveness through clinical studies.

FDA may take any of the following actions on a 510(k) after conducting its review (21 CFR § 807.100(a)): find the device substantially equivalent to the predicate and issue a clearance letter, find the device not substantially equivalent (NSE) and issue an NSE letter prohibiting marketing, or request additional information (with the final clearance decision pending review of that information). A manufacturer generally has 30 days to provide any additional information, or FDA may issue a notice of withdrawal of the application (21 CFR § 807.87(l)). The manufacturer may, at any time, withdraw its 510(k). FDA has 90 days to review a traditional 510(k).[37]

Abbreviated and special 510(k)s were new approaches to premarket notification that came from FDAMA of 1997, intended to streamline and expedite FDA's review for routine submissions meeting certain qualifications, thus leaving more reviewer time for more complicated submissions. An abbreviated 510(k) uses guidance documents developed by FDA to communicate regulatory and scientific expectations to industry. Guidance documents have been prepared for many different kinds of devices, and are available on FDA's website. All guidance documents are developed in accordance with Good Guidance Practices (GGP, 21 CFR § 10.115)), and many with public participation or opportunities for public comment.[38]

In addition to issuing guidance documents, FDA can either develop performance or consensus standards or 'recognize' those developed by outside parties (21 CFR Part 861). In an abbreviated 510(k), the manufacturer describes what guidance document, special control, or performance standard was used, and how it was used to assess performance of their device.

Other minimum required elements are the product description, representative labeling, and a summary of the performance characteristics. FDA typically reviews an abbreviated 510(k) in 60 days.

The Quality System Regulation (QSR; 21 CFR § 820.30) is the regulation that describes the good manufacturing practice (GMP) requirements for medical devices (see the Manufacturing section of this report for more detail on QSR). A special 510(k) utilizes the design control[39] requirement of the QSR and may be used for a modification to a device that has already been cleared. The modifications should not affect the safety and effectiveness of the device. The special 510(k) allows the manufacturer to declare conformance to design controls, without providing the data. This type of submission references the original 510(k) number, and contains information about the design control requirements. FDA aims to review most special 510(k)s in 30 days.

Under the FFDCA, novel devices lacking a legally marketed predicate would automatically be designated Class III. FDAMA amended Section 513(f) to allow FDA to establish a new, expedited mechanism for reclassifying these devices based on risk, thus reducing the regulatory burden on manufacturers. The de novo 510(k), though requiring more data than a traditional 510(k), often requires less information than a premarket application (PMA), discussed below.

In a *de novo* 510(k) process, the manufacturer submits a traditional 510(k) for its device. However, because there is no predicate device or classification, the agency will return a decision of not substantially equivalent. Within 30 days, the manufacturer submits a petition requesting reclassification of its device into Class II or I, as appropriate. Within 60 days, FDA will render a decision classifying the device according to criteria in 51 3(a)(1) of FFDCA. With approval, FDA issues a regulation that classifies the device. If the device is Class II, a special controls guidance document is also developed that then allows subsequent manufacturers to submit either traditional or abbreviated 510(k)s.[40]

Premarket Application (PMA)

A PMA is the most stringent type of device marketing application required by FDA for new and/or high-risk devices. PMA approval is based on a determination by FDA that the application contains sufficient valid scientific evidence to assure that the device is safe and effective for its intended use(s) (21 CFR Part 814). A PMA must contain the following information (among other things): administrative requirements, summaries of non-clinical and clinical data supporting the intended use and performance characteristics, detailed information on the design of the device and a description of the device components, instructions for use, representations of packaging and labeling, a description of means by which users can assess the quality of the device, information about any computer software or additional or special equipment needed, literature about the disease and the similar devices, information on the manufacturing process, and assurance of compliance with QSR.

In contrast to a 510(k), PMAs generally require some clinical data, but can also use studies from the medical literature (a "paper PMA"). Approval is based not only on the strength of the scientific data, but also on inspection of the manufacturing facility to assure that the facility and the manufacturing process are in compliance with the quality systems regulations (QSR: 21 CFR Part 820). FDAMA made it easier for manufacturers to submit the required sections of a PMA in a serial fashion as data are available ("modular PMA").

When a PMA is first received, FDA has 45 days to make sure the application is administratively complete. If so, FDA formally files the application. If not, the application is returned. FDA then has 75 days to complete the initial review and determine whether an advisory committee meeting will be necessary.

Advisory committees, comprised of scientific, medical, and statistical experts, and industry and consumer representatives, can be convened to make recommendations on any scientific or policy matter before FDA.[41] They allow for interested persons to present information and views at an oral public hearing before the advisory committee (21 CFR Part 14). FDA typically accepts advisory committee recommendations for an application (approvable, approvable with conditions or non-approvable); however, there have been cases where the decision has not been consistent with the recommendation (e.g., where the conditions for approval are so burdensome as to practically present a non-approvable situation). CDRH will hold joint advisory committee meetings with other centers where necessary.

After FDA notifies the applicant that the PMA has been approved or denied, a notice may be published on the Internet (1) announcing the data on which the decision is based, and (2) providing interested persons an opportunity to petition FDA within 30 days for reconsideration of the decision. Though FDA regulations allow 180 days to review the PMA and make a determination (21 CFR § 814.40), in reality the review time could be much longer. Pursuant to MDUFMA and FDAAA performance goals have been established to reduce the review time for PMAs.

Supplements to 510(k)s and PMAs

Once a device has been cleared through a 510(k) process or approved through the PMA process, the manufacturer can market the device only for the intended use that FDA cleared or approved. For example, a device, such as a stent, approved to treat coronary artery disease may not be marketed for treatment of blocked biliary ducts unless the manufacturer files additional information with FDA to demonstrate that the device is safe and effective for the new use. The information can be filed as a supplement to the original application. Supplements are required not only for new uses of a cleared or approved device, but also for design or manufacturing changes that may impact safety and effectiveness (e.g., changing the type of metal or plastic on a device, or using a different antibody for diagnosis of a disease).

Investigational Device Exemption (IDE)

An IDE allows an unapproved device (most commonly an invasive or life-sustaining device) to be used in a clinical study to collect data required to support a submission, most commonly a PMA, at some later point in time.[42] Investigational use can also include clinical evaluation of certain modifications to or new intended uses of legally marketed devices (e.g., supplemental application). All clinical evaluations of investigational devices, unless they are exempt, must have an IDE and be approved by an institutional review board (IRB), before the study is initiated.[43] The IDE permits a device to be shipped lawfully for investigation of the device without requiring that the manufacturer comply with other requirements of the FFDCA, such as registration and listing. Manufacturers of devices with IDE's are also exempt from the quality systems regulations (QSR), except for the requirements for design control.

While under investigation, manufacturers, sponsors, clinical investigators and IRBs must comply with Good Clinical Practices, including all regulations that govern the conduct of clinical studies:

Investigational Device Exemptions (21 CFR Part 812) covering the procedures for the conduct of clinical studies with medical devices including application, responsibilities of sponsors and investigators, labeling, records, and reports;
Protection of Human Subjects (21 CFR Part 50) providing the requirements and general elements of informed consent;
Institutional Review Boards (21 CFR Part 56) covering the procedures and responsibilities for IRBs that approve clinical investigations protocols;
Financial Disclosure by Clinical Investigators (21 CFR Part 54) covering the disclosure of financial compensation to clinical investigators which is part of FDA's assessment of the reliability of the clinical data; and
Design Controls of the QSR (21 CFR Part 820 Subpart C) providing the requirement for procedures to control the design of the device in order to ensure that the specified design requirements are met.

Devices are exempt from IDE requirements when testing is noninvasive, does not require invasive sampling, does not introduce energy into a subject, and is not stand alone (i.e., is not used for diagnosis without confirmation by other methods or medically established procedures) (21 CFR § 812.2(c)(3)).

Humanitarian Device Exemption (HDE)

An HDE is an application that is similar to a PMA, but exempt from the effectiveness requirements. An approved HDE authorizes marketing of a humanitarian use device. A humanitarian use device is intended to benefit patients in the treatment and diagnosis of diseases or conditions that affect fewer than 4,000 individuals in the U.S. per year. The exemption from proving effectiveness is designed to encourage manufacturers to develop medical devices for these small markets, assisting patients with rare diseases and conditions who might otherwise not be served.

Before submitting an HDE application, the manufacturer submits a request for a humanitarian use device designation to FDA's Office of Orphan Products Development (OOPD). The request includes (1) a statement that they are requesting a humanitarian use device designation for a rare disease or condition; (2) the name and address of the manufacturer; (3) a description of the rare disease or condition for which the device is to be used; (4) a description of the device; and (5) documentation, with appended authoritative references, to demonstrate that the device is designed to treat or diagnose a disease or condition that affects or is manifested in fewer than 4,000 people in the United States per year (see 21 CFR § 814.102(a)). In order for a device to receive marketing approval under this regulation, there should not be another legally marketed device available to treat or diagnose the disease or condition. Once a device with the same intended use as the humanitarian use device is approved or cleared, an HDE cannot be granted for the humanitarian use device.

The agency has 75 days from the date of receipt to review an HDE application. This includes a 30-day filing period during which the agency determines whether the HDE application is sufficiently complete to permit substantive review. FDA does require that a manufacturer comply with the QSR that the agency deems most relevant to the safety of the device. Alternatively, the manufacturer can request an exemption. Supplements, and sometimes even a new HDE, are required for additional indications.[44]

In Vitro Diagnostic Products (IVD)

IVD products are "... those reagents, instruments, and systems intended for use in diagnosis of disease or other conditions, including a determination of the state of health, in order to cure, mitigate, treat, or prevent disease or its sequelae. Such products are intended for use in the collection, preparation, and examination of specimens taken from the human body (21 CFR § 809.3). IVDs are medical devices as defined in Section 210(h) of the FFDCA (such as gene chips), and may also be biological products subject to Section 351 of the Public Health Service Act (such as biological agent diagnostic systems).

IVDs are different from other medical devices in that they do not act directly on a patient to produce a result like an implantable, life-sustaining or other device does. Instead, the risk to the patient is from the generation of inaccurate test results (i.e., wrong answers) that lead to mismanagement of a patient's condition.

IVDs (e.g., laboratory tests) may consist of general purpose reagents,[45] analyte specific reagents (ASRs),[46] general purpose or specific equipment, sometimes with computer analysis software.[47] Most stand-alone items of general purpose equipment, such as automated clinical analyzers, are exempt Class I devices. However, if the equipment performs a specific test, equipment plus the test becomes a test system. Test systems are considered combination devices, and they are classified according to the risk level of the highest of the two device classifications (i.e., an analyzer may be Class I exempt, but if a manufacturer wishes to market it with an HIV test kit, the system could be regulated as a Class III device and require a PMA). Most IVD products are reviewed in CDRH's Office of In Vitro Diagnostic Device Evaluation and Safety (OIVD), and CBER's Office of Blood Research and Review (OBRR). The classification of existing IVDs can be found in 21 CFR Part 862, 21 CFR Part 864, and 21 CFR Part 866.

Like other medical devices, IVDs are subject to premarket and postmarket controls. But unlike other devices, IVDs are also subject to the Clinical Laboratory Improvement Amendments (CLIA) of 1988.[48] CLIA establishes quality standards for laboratory testing and an accreditation program for clinical laboratories that perform testing using IVD products. CLIA requirements vary according to the technical complexity in the testing process and risk of harm in reporting erroneous results. The regulations establish three categories of testing on the basis of the complexity of the testing methodology: (a) waived tests, (b) tests of moderate complexity, and (c) tests of high complexity.

Manufacturers apply for CLIA categorization (determined by FDA)[49] during the premarket process. Postmarket, the Centers for Medicare and Medicaid Services (CMS) regulates all laboratory testing (except research) performed on humans in the U.S. through CLIA.[50] Under CLIA, laboratories performing only waived tests are subject to minimal regulation. Laboratories performing moderate or high complexity tests are subject to specific laboratory standards governing certification, personnel, proficiency testing, patient test management, quality assurance, quality control, and inspections.

CLIA categorization (defining regulatory requirements on the laboratory testing process) do not always match FDA classification (defining regulatory requirements on the tests kits or systems themselves). For example, a "waived" test under CLIA is the simplest test to perform (usually by an untrained user), with the smallest margin of error. As such, they receive little to no oversight under CLIA. However, FDA may designate such a test as Class III, so that it undergoes rigorous review to insure that it performs as advertised (i.e., with a small margin of error in the hands of an untrained user).

Most IVDs are exempt from IDE requirements. Because the benefits and risks to the patient from use of IVDs are indirect (i.e., due to the use of the test result in patient management), FDA requires that the companies demonstrate analytical test performance in patient samples that would test along the continuum of positive and negative for the marker of interest. In addition, FDA requires support for the clinical validity of the test (i.e., evidence that the biological marker that the test is detecting actually is associated with the disease or condition that the company wishes to market the test for in a predictable way).

For some of the applications seeking clearance for an IVD, biological markers that the test purports to measure may be relatively well characterized with respect to a disease and patient population (such as the link between glucose measurement and diabetes). In these cases, analytical studies using clinically derived samples (e.g., blood specimens from healthy and diabetic individuals) suffice to show that the test is actually detecting the marker. Sometimes clinical samples can be supplemented by carefully selected artificial samples, particularly if a disease, condition or marker is rare. For example, if FDA were to review a genetic test to measure genetic markers for drug metabolism, they may require the manufacturer to use actual patient samples to demonstrate that they can detect common markers. FDA may, however, allow the company to use artificial or 'spiked' samples to test for rare markers so that the company would not have to test an overly burdensome number of clinical samples. In this type of submission, the manufacturer could use medical literature to support the clinical validity of the biological marker to the disease, and would not have to conduct a clinical study to demonstrate that the test measures the marker and the marker is associated with the disease.

For other IVDs, the link between analytical performance of the test in its ability to detect a biological marker and the clinical validity of the marker is not well defined. In these circumstances, new clinical information may be required. FDA rarely requires prospective clinical studies for IVDs, but regularly requests clinical samples with sufficient laboratory and/or clinical characterization to allow an assessment of the clinical validity of a new device. For example, a company seeking to market a test for a new tumor marker may use well-characterized, archived patient samples collected as part of a completely separate study to demonstrate that their test can classify patients in a predictable way. Clinical performance is usually expressed in terms of clinical sensitivity and clinical specificity (when compared to a disease or health state) or agreement (when compared to performance of a predicate device or reference method). For most PMAs, manufacturers identify surrogate endpoints (such as tumor shrinking or reduction in a tumor marker) and establish the device performance in relation to those rather than to disease outcome (such as improved survival).

THE MEDICAL DEVICE APPROVAL PROCESS: POST-APPROVAL REQUIREMENTS AND ISSUES

Once approved or cleared for marketing, manufacturers of medical devices must comply with regulations on labeling and advertising, on production of their device, and on postmarket surveillance of adverse events associated with the use of their device. The requirements for each of these are described below.

Labeling

Like drugs and biological products, all FDA approved or cleared medical devices are required to be labeled in a way that informs a user of how to use the device in a safe and effective manner. Section 201(k) of the FFDCA defines a "label" as a: "display of written, printed, or graphic matter upon the immediate container of any article." Section 201(m) defines "labeling" as: "all labels and other written, printed, or graphic matter upon any article or any of its containers or wrappers, or accompanying such article" at any time while a device is held for sale after shipment or delivery for shipment in interstate commerce. The term "accompanying" is interpreted to mean more than physical association with the product; it extends to posters, tags, pamphlets, circulars, booklets, brochures, instruction books, direction sheets, fillers, webpages, etc. "Accompanying can also include labeling that is connected with the device after shipment or delivery for shipment in interstate commerce. According to an appellate court decision "Most, if not all advertising, is labeling. The term 'labeling' is defined in the FFDCA as including all printed matter accompanying any article. Congress did not, and we cannot, exclude from the definition printed matter which constitutes advertising."[51]

Labeling regulations pertaining to medical devices are found in the following parts of Title 21 CFR:

General Device Labeling (21 CFR Part 801)
In Vitro Diagnostic Products (21 CFR Part 809)
Investigational Device Exemptions (21 CFR Part 812)
Good Manufacturing Practices (21 CFR Part 820)
General Electronic Products (21 CFR Part 1010)

All devices must conform to the general labeling requirements. Certain devices[52] require specific labeling which may include not only package labeling, but informational literature, patient release forms, performance testing, and/or specific tolerances or prohibitions on certain ingredients.

Various sections of the QSR have an impact on labeling: Section 21 CFR § 820.80(b) requires the inspection and testing of incoming materials including labeling; and 21 CFR § 820.70(f) requires buildings to be of suitable design and have sufficient space for packaging and labeling operations; 21 CFR § 820.120 deals with specific requirements for the control of labeling. This regulation applies to the application of labeling to ensure legibility under normal conditions of use over the expected life of the device; and also applies to inspection, handling, storage, and distribution of labeling. FDA considers a device to be adulterated if these requirements are not met. These requirements do not apply to the adequacy of labeling content, except to make sure the content meets labeling specifications contained in the device master record. However, failure to comply with GMP requirements, such as proofreading and change control, could result in labeling content errors. In such cases, the device could be misbranded and/or adulterated.

Manufacturing

Like drug manufacturers, medical device manufacturers must produce their devices in accordance with Good Manufacturing Practice (GMP). The GMP requirements for devices are described in the QSR, (FFDCA §520; 21 CFR 820). The QSRs require that domestic or foreign manufacturers have a quality system for the design, manufacture, packaging, labeling, storage, installation, and servicing of non-exempt finished medical devices intended for commercial distribution in the United States. The regulation requires that various specifications and controls be established for devices; that devices be designed and manufactured under a quality system to meet these specifications; that finished devices meet these specifications; that devices be correctly installed, checked and serviced; that quality data be analyzed to identify and correct quality problems; and that complaints be processed. FDA monitors device problem data and inspects the operations and records of device developers and manufacturers to determine compliance with the GMP requirements.[53]

Though FDA has identified in QSR the essential elements that a quality system should have, manufacturers have a great deal of leeway to design quality systems that best cover nuances of their devices and the means of producing them.

Postmarket Surveillance

Once their device is approved or cleared, manufacturers must conduct postmarket surveillance studies to gather safety and efficacy data for certain devices introduced into interstate commerce after January 1, 1991. This requirement applies to devices that

> are permanent implants, the failure of which may cause serious adverse health consequences or death;
> are intended for use in supporting or sustaining human life; or
> present a potential serious risk to human health.

FDA may require postmarket surveillance for other devices if deemed necessary to protect the public health. The primary objective of postmarket surveillance is to study the performance of the device after clearance or approval as it is used in the population for which it is intended—and to discover cases of device failure and its attendant impact on the patient.

Manufacturers may receive notification that their device is subject to postmarket surveillance when FDA files (i.e., accepts) the submission, and again when a final decision is made. If notified, manufacturers must submit a plan for postmarket surveillance to FDA for approval within 30 days of introducing their device into interstate commerce.

MDUFMA authorized additional appropriations for postmarket surveillance—$3 million for FY2003, $6 million for FY2004, and such sums as may be necessary in subsequent years; however, the money was not appropriated. FDAAA authorized the appropriation of $25 million per year for Postmarket Studies and Surveillance (21 USC 355 note).

Adverse Event Reporting

Section 519(a) of the FFDCA as amended by the SMDA of 1990 required FDA to establish a system for monitoring and tracking serious adverse events that resulted from the use or misuse of medical devices. The Medical Device Reporting (MDR) regulation is the mechanism that FDA and manufacturers use to identify and monitor significant adverse events involving medical devices, so that problems are detected and corrected in a timely manner. User facilities (e.g., hospitals, nursing homes, clinical laboratories) are required to report suspected medical device- related deaths to both FDA and the manufacturers within 10 working days. User facilities may report medical device related serious injuries only to the manufacturer within 10 days. Manufacturers must file a summary of all medical device reports to FDA within 30 calendar days. User facilities must file a summary report annually. Although the FFDCA gives FDA the authority to impose legal sanctions for not complying with MDR, FDA relies largely on the goodwill and cooperation of all affected groups to accomplish the objectives of the regulation.

Medical Device Tracking

Manufacturers must adopt a method of tracking certain devices. These are devices:

whose failurc would be reasonably likely to have serious, adverse health consequences; or
which are intended to be implanted in the human body for more than one year; or
which are life-sustaining or life-supporting devices used outside of a device user facility (21 CFR Part 821).

The purpose of device tracking is to ensure that manufacturers of these devices can locate them quickly once in commercial distribution if needed to facilitate notifications and recalls in the case of serious risks to health presented by the devices.[54]

Compliance and Enforcement

Compliance requirements apply to both the premarket approval process and postmarket surveillance. When a problem arises with a product regulated by FDA, the agency can take a number of actions to protect the public health. Initially, the agency tries to work with the manufacturer to correct the problem on a voluntary basis. If that fails, legal remedies may be taken, such as: asking the manufacturer to recall a product, having federal marshals seize products, or detaining imports at the port of entry until problems are corrected. If warranted, FDA can ask the courts to issue injunctions or prosecute individual company officers that deliberately violate the law. When warranted, criminal penalties, including prison sentences, may be sought.

Each center has an Office of Compliance (OC) which ensures compliance with regulations while pre- or postmarket studies are being undertaken, with manufacturing requirements, and with labeling requirements. The objectives of CDRH's OC's Bioresearch Monitoring (BIMO) program are to ensure the quality and integrity of data and information submitted in support of IDE, PMA, and 510(k) submissions and to ensure that human subjects taking part in investigations are protected from undue hazard or risk. This is achieved through audits of clinical data contained in PMAs prior to approval, data audits of IDE and 510(k) submissions, inspections of IRBs and nonclinical laboratories, and enforcement of the prohibitions against promotion, marketing, or commercialization of investigational devices. Any establishment where devices are manufactured, processed, packed, installed, used, or implanted or where records of results from use of devices are kept, can be subject to inspection.

The OC also reviews the quality system design and manufacturing information in the PMA submission to determine whether the manufacturer has described the processes in sufficient detail and to make a preliminary determination of whether the manufacturer meets the QSR. If the manufacturer has provided an adequate description of the design and manufacturing process, a preapproval inspection can be initiated. Inspection is to include an assessment of the manufacturer's capability to design and manufacture the device as claimed in the PMA and confirm that the quality system is in compliance with the QSR. Postapproval inspections can be conducted within eight to twelve months of approval of the PMA submission. The inspection is to primarily focus on any changes that may have been made in the device design, manufacturing process, or quality systems.

The compliance offices work closely with the Office of Regulatory Affairs (ORA),[55] which operates in the field to regulate almost 124,000 business establishments that annually produce, warehouse, import and transport $1 trillion worth of medical products. Consumer safety officers (CSOs) and inspectors typically have conducted about 22,000 domestic and foreign inspections a year to ensure that regulated products meet the agency's standards. CSOs also monitor clinical trials. Scientists in ORA's 13 laboratories typically have analyzed more than 41,000 product samples each year to determine their adherence to FDA's standards.

Section 516 of the FFDCA gives FDA the authority to ban devices that present substantial deception or unreasonable and substantial risk of illness or injury. Section 518 enables FDA to require manufacturers or other appropriate individuals to notify all health professionals who prescribe or use the device and any other person (including manufacturers, importers, distributors, retailers, and device users) of any health risks resulting from the use of a violative device, so that these risks may be reduced or eliminated. This section also gives consumers a procedure for economic redress when they have been sold defective medical devices that present unreasonable risks. Section 519 of the act authorized FDA to promulgate regulations requiring manufacturers, importers, and distributors of devices to maintain records and reports to assure that devices are not adulterated or misbranded. Section 5 20(e) of the MDA authorized FDA to restrict the sale, distribution, or use of a device if there cannot otherwise be reasonable assurance of its safety and effectiveness. A restricted device can only be sold on oral or written authorization by a licensed practitioner or under conditions specified by regulation.

Warning Letter

A warning letter is a written communication from FDA notifying a responsible individual, manufacturer, or facility that the agency considers one or more products, practices, processes, or other activities to be in violation of the laws that FDA enforces. The warning letter informs the recipient that failure to take appropriate and prompt action to correct and prevent any future repeat of the violations could result in an administrative or regulatory action. Although serious noncompliance is often a catalyst for issuance of a warning letter, the warning letter is informal and advisory.

A congressional report found the CDRH issued 65% fewer such warning letters in 2005 than in 2000, although the number of violations by food and drug manufacturers observed by FDA agents during field inspections has remained relatively constant.[56] The report suggested that the lack of enforcement actions may have been due in part to FDA officials rejecting FDA field inspectors enforcement recommendations. FDA's Office of Legislation offered an alternative explanation, referencing a change in policy related to a specific program—the Mammography Quality Standards Act (MQSA, P.L. 102-539) (see **Table 3**).

Product Recall

A recall is a method of removing or correcting products that FDA considers are in violation of the law.[57] Medical device recalls are usually conducted voluntarily by the manufacturer (21 CFR Part 7), after negotiation with FDA. Under 21 CFR Part 806, manufacturers (including refurbishers and reconditioners) and importers are required to report to FDA any correction or removal of a medical device that is undertaken to reduce a health risk posed by the device. A recall may be a total market withdrawal or may be of a portion of product (such as a single lot). In rare instances, where the manufacturer or importer fails to voluntarily recall a device that is a risk to health, FDA may issue a recall order to the manufacturer (21 CFR Part 81 0).[58]

When a recall is initiated, FDA performs an evaluation of the health hazard presented taking into account the following factors, among others:

> Whether any disease or injuries have already occurred from the use of the product;
> Whether any existing conditions could contribute to a clinical situation that could expose humans or animals to a health hazard;
> Assessment of hazard to various segments of the population, (e.g., children, surgical patients, pets, livestock, etc.), who would be exposed to the product;
> Assessment of the degree of seriousness of the health hazard to which the populations at risk would be exposed;
> Assessment of the likelihood of occurrence of the hazard;
> Assessment of the consequences (immediate or long-range) of occurrence of the hazard.

Following the health hazard assessment, FDA assigns the recall a classification according to the relative degree of health hazard. *Class I* recalls are the most serious, reserved for situations where there is a reasonable probability that the use of, or exposure to, a product will cause serious adverse health consequences or death. *Class II* recalls are for situations where the use of, or exposure to, a product may cause temporary or medically reversible adverse health consequences or where the probability of serious adverse health consequences is remote. In a *Class III* recall situation, the use of, or exposure to, a product is not likely to cause adverse health consequences.

In addition to a warning letter or recall, FDA may also issue a public notification or safety alert (e.g., "Dear Doctor" letter), to warn healthcare providers and consumers of the risk of the device in question.

Table 3. CDRH Warning Letters Issued in Total and Under the MQSA, FY2000-FY2008

	Non-MQSA	MQSA	Total
FY2000	191	337	528
FY2001	105	393	498
FY2002	75	206	285
FY2003	121	84	205
FY2004	193	5	198
FY2005	177	5	182
FY2006	149	5	154
FY2007	146	10	52
FY2008	164	2	166

Source: FDA Office of Legislation.

Notes: According to FDA's Office of Legislation, the number of MQSA warning letters has significantly decreased because of a change in ORA and CDRH policy. Enforcement strategies for violations of the MQSA now focus on opportunities for correction and re-inspections (fees paid by facilities) prior to issuing warning letters. These measures have reduced the number of warning letters the program has had to issue.

LEGISLATION

A number of medical device related topics are of interest to members of the 111th Congress. As described below, these include 510(k) clearance, liability and preemption, medicare and other federal coverage, importation, advertising, IVD regulation, and some other issues.

Liability and Preemption

Two recent United States Supreme Court cases focus on the question of whether FDA approval protects a manufacturer from liability under state tort law.[59] The first case, *Riegel v. Medtronic, Inc.*, involved an FDA-approved medical device.[60] In *Riegel*, the Supreme Court held that if the FDA grants a PMA for a medical device, the device manufacturer is immune from suit under state common law claims such as strict liability, breach of implied warranty, and negligence in design, testing, labeling, manufacturing, labeling, distribution, sale, inspection, or marketing of the device. The court's holding in *Riegel* suggests that FDA approval prevents consumers from suing manufacturers in some circumstances. In other words, it suggests preemption rather than liability.

By contrast, the second case, *Wyeth v. Levine*, which dealt with an FDA-approved drug, suggests that FDA approval does not prevent consumers from suing under state law. [61] In other words, it suggests liability rather than preemption. In *Wyeth,* the Supreme Court held that FDA's approval of a drug does not preempt a lawsuit against the manufacturer alleging that the drug's label failed to provide an adequate warning against significant risks. The court drew a distinction between *Riegel* and *Wyeth* based on differences in congressional action regarding drugs and devices: "when Congress enacted an express pre-emption provision for medical devices in 1976, see §521, 90 Stat. 574 (codified at 21 U. S. C. §360k(a)), it declined to enact such a provision for prescription drugs."

Some members of Congress have proposed legislation on the topic of what effect, if any, FDA approval should have on a manufacturer's liability.

510(k) Clearance

FDAAA (the FDA Amendments Act of 2007) required the Government Accountability Office (GAO) to study and report on the appropriate use of the 510(k) process to determine whether a new device is as safe and effective as a classified device.[62] The report, released in January 2009, made one recommendation: that FDA expeditiously take steps to issue regulations for class III device types currently allowed to enter the market via the 510(k) process (i.e., preamendment devices) by requiring PMAs or reclassifying them to a lower class. [63] The report has sparked a range of legislative interest in issues related to 510(k) and preamendment devices.

Medicare and Other Federal Coverage

While FDA does not generally consider or regulate the cost of medical devices,[64] the way that medical devices are reimbursed in the public health care system is of interest to many members of Congress.[65] Some members have focused on measures to help keep prices low, such as requiring the reporting of sales price data for certain devices. Others have sought to enhance access by amending payment formulas, requiring for Medicare coverage for FDA approved devices, or eliminating certain preconditions for payment. Issues related to the cost of medical products are also of potential relevance to legislative discussions focused on health care reform and cost effectiveness.

Importation and Inspection

FDA shares its responsibility for ensuring the safety of imported medical devices with other agencies, including Customs and Border Protection. Questions raised about the safety of imported medical products have led some members of Congress to propose requiring enhanced registration for manufacturers and other establishments, the identification of prior transactions in device production, country of manufacture labeling, the hire of additional foreign inspectors, risk-based inspection, and other measures.

Advertising

FDA has the authority to regulate the advertising of *restricted* medical devices, which are the rough equivalent of *prescription* drugs (FFDCA 5 02(r)). (The Federal Trade Commission regulates the marketing of non-restricted devices.) On one hand, advertising to consumers and health professionals might serve to educate them about life enhancing products. On the other, it might bias them, and raise device prices by the amount of advertising costs. Members of Congress have proposed legislation to regulate how medical device companies should promote their devices to consumers and physicians, as well as to require disclosure of companies' gifts to physicians.

IVD Regulation

FDA claims the authority to regulate all laboratory tests; however, it does not regulate all IVDs.[66] Whether FDA regulates a test depends on whether it is a laboratory-developed test (i.e., developed in-house, not for commercial distribution, also known as home brews) or a kit intended for commercial distribution. FDA regulates tests that are kits, and it does not regulate lab- developed tests in their entirety. (Certain components of lab-developed tests, called analyte specific reagents, are regulated by the FDA as Class I devices if they are commercially distributed.) While some argue that less regulation of laboratory developed tests aids consumer access to rapidly developed personalized tests, others argue that more regulation would help to ensure that the tests are accurate. Some members of Congress have proposed legislative measures that address the topic of IVD regulation.

Other Issues

Medical devices are relevant to some other topics of legislative interest as well, such as efforts to make transparent the exchange of payment or other transfer of value between manufacturers and physicians,[67] prohibit the use of live animals for marketing medical devices,[68] or to ease restrictions the exportation to Cuba of medical devices and other products.[69]

End Notes

[1] PriceWaterhouseCoopers/ National Venture Capital Association, "Medical Devices and Equipment," *Money Tree Report*, data provided by Thomson Reuters searched December 29, 2008.
[2] Global Insight, "Venture Impact: The Economic Importance of Venture Capital Backed Companies to the U.S. Economy, Fourth Edition" (2008)

[3] See "Maryland Hospital Officials Resign After Patients Receive Incorrect HIV, Hepatitis C Test Results Processed in Lab," *Kaiser Network, Across The Nation* (April 22, 2004)

[4] See "Medical Device Recalls, Class I Recall: Boston Scientific Express Coronary Stent," "Medical Device Recalls, Class I Recall: Boston Scientific Taxus Express Coronary Stent," and "Medical Device Recalls, Class 1 Recall: Access CardioSystems Automated External Defibrillators,"

[5] FDA, "Devices Regulated by CBER," (updated March 15, 2007)

[6] For more information on FDA's budget, See CRS Report RL34334, *The Food and Drug Administration: Budget and Statutory History, FY1980-FY2007*, coordinated by Judith A. Johnson; and CRS Report RL34638, *FDA FY2009 Appropriations*, by Susan Thaul et al.

[7] For more information about medical device user fees, see CRS Report RL34571, *Medical Device User Fees and User Fee Acts*, by Erin D. Williams, and CRS Report RL33981, *Medical Device User Fee and Modernization Act (MDUFMA) Reauthorization*, by Erin D. Williams. FDA also funds some device and radiological health activities with fees collected under the Mammography Quality Standards Act (MQSA, P.L. 102-539).

[8] See CRS Report RS22946, *Food and Drug Administration (FDA): Overview and Issues*, by Erin D. Williams.

[9] See CRS Report RL34465, *FDA Amendments Act of 2007 (P.L. 110-85)*, by Erin D. Williams and Susan Thaul.

[10] See CRS Report RL34334, *The Food and Drug Administration: Budget and Statutory History, FY1980-FY2007*, coordinated by Judith A. Johnson, and CRS Report RL34638, *FDA FY2009 Appropriations*, by Susan Thaul et al.

[11] Union of Concerned Scientists "Voices of Scientists at FDA: Protecting Public Health Depends on Independent Science," 2006,

[12] For example, Senator Grassley expressed dissatisfaction with FDA's lack of responsiveness and transparency. "Grassley questions FDA about risks to children, infants in antibiotic drug trials," *Senator Chuck Grassley Press Release* (June 8, 2008), at http://grassley.senate.gov/index.cfm?FuseAction=PressReleases.Detail&PressRelease_id=5092&Month=6&Year=2006. A Congressional report characterized FDA's answers to requests for information as haphazard, incomplete, and untimely. United States House of Representatives Committee on Government Reform Minority Staff, Prescription for Harm: The Decline in FDA Enforcement Activity, Special Investigation prepared for Representative Henry A. Waxman (June 2006), p. 4

[13] Federal Food, Drug and Cosmetic Act §201(h), (21 U.S.C. 321)

[14] The Lewin Group, for AdvaMed, *The Impact of Regulation and Market Dynamics on Innovation: The State of the Industry* (Washington, DC, 2001).

[15] Frost & Sullivan estimate in Robert Gold, "Healthcare: Products & Supplies, Industry Profile," *Standard and Poor's Industry Survey*, September 18, 2008; and Herman Saftlas, "Healthcare: Pharmaceuticals, Industry Profile," *Standard and Poor's Industry Survey*, April 24, 2008.

[16] See CRS Report RL34571, *Medical Device User Fees and User Fee Acts*, by Erin D. Williams; For historical background, see CRS Report RL33981, *Medical Device User Fee and Modernization Act (MDUFMA) Reauthorization*, by Erin D. Williams.

[17] See CRS Report RL34465, *FDA Amendments Act of 2007 (P.L. 110-85)*, by Erin D. Williams and Susan Thaul.

[18] See CRS Report RL32832, *Clinical Trials Reporting and Publication*, by Erin D. Williams.

[19] FDA uses advisory committees to gain independent advice from outside experts. See CRS Report RS22691, *FDA Advisory Committee Conflict of Interest*, by Erin D. Williams.

[20] The term *manufacturer* is used throughout this report for simplicity, but regulations also apply to any person, organization, or sponsor that submits an application to FDA to market a device.

[21] Certain medical devices that present only a minimal risk, such as plastic bandages and ice bags, can be legally marketed upon registration alone. These low-risk devices are deemed *exempt* from premarket review, and manufacturers need not submit an application to FDA prior to marketing them. Manufacturers of exempt devices are still typically required to comply with other regulations, known as general controls. (21 CFR 862-892).

[22] 21 CFR § 860.7(c)(2).

[23] 21 CFR § 860.7(d)(1).

[24] 21 CFR § 860.7(d)(2).

[25] 21 CFR § 860.7(e)(1).

[26] To be a predicate, a device must have either been on the market before 1976 when the MDA took effect, or it could have been cleared for marketing after 1976, but must have the same intended use as a device classified in the CFR.

[27] The statement of intended use is a general description of the diseases or conditions that the device will diagnose, treat, prevent, cure, or mitigate, including a description, where appropriate, of the patient population for which the device is intended. (21 CFR § 807.92(a)(5), and § 814.20 (b)(3)(I))

[28] Preamendment medical devices (those on the market prior to the passage of the MDA in 1976) were presumed to be marketable. They did not need to undergo premarket review, and could be legally unless and until FDA required their removal. As required by the MDA, FDA classified the preamendment devices and used them as

the basis for creating the classification panels and as the first cadre of predicate devices that could be used to demonstrate substantial equivalence.

[29] The term "manufacturer" is used throughout this report for simplicity, but also includes any person, organization, or sponsor that submits a marketing application to FDA for marketing approval for a medical device.

[30] FFDCA 513(a)(1)(A); also see FDA, *General Controls for Medical Devices*, April 16, 1998

[31] See CRS Report RL34571, *Medical Device User Fees and User Fee Acts*, by Erin D. Williams.

[32] A device is adulterated if it includes any filthy, putrid, or decomposed substance, or if it is prepared, packed, or held under unsanitary conditions. The FDC Act further states that a device is adulterated if its container contains any poisonous or deleterious substance, or if its strength, purity or quality varies significantly from what the manufacturer claims. For higher class devices, a device can be considered adulterated if it fails to meet performance requirements outlined in its approval, or if it is in violation of other Good Manufacturing Practice requirements.

[33] A device is misbranded when all or part of the labeling (i.e., the FDA-approved printed material providing information about the device) is false, misleading, or missing.

[34] For guidance on the procedures established, see *Early Collaboration Meetings Under the FDA Modernization Act*; Final Guidance for Industry and CDRH Staff, February 28, 2001

[35] For more information on the IDE, please refer to the "Marketing Applications for Medical Devices" section that immediately follows this discussion.

[36] FDA, "Content of a 510(k)," June 30, 2003 and *How to Prepare a Traditional 510(k)*, January 4, 2005

[37] The FDA time clock (i.e., review cycle) begins when FDA receives the 5 10(k) and ends with the date that FDA issues either a request for additional information or a decision. More than one cycle may occur before FDA issues its final decision.

[38] FDA continually accepts public comment on any draft or final guidance document.

[39] Design controls are a series of predetermined checks, verifications, and specifications that are built into the manufacturing process to validate the quality of the product throughout the process. These can include defining the personnel responsible for implementing steps in the development and manufacturing process, defining specifications and standards for assessing the quality of the materials that go into making the product, designing specifications for accepting and rejecting different batches or lots of final product, and requirements for maintaining appropriate records.

[40] Guidance for Industry and FDA Staff, New Section 513(f)(2)—*Evaluation of Automatic Class III Designation*, February 19, 1998

[41] For further information, see CRS Report RS22691, *FDA Advisory Committee Conflict of Interest*, by Erin D. Williams.

[42] FDA, IDE Overview, July 8, 2003

[43] An IRB is a group, generally comprised volunteers, that examines proposed and ongoing scientific research to ensure that human subjects are properly protected. For further information, see CRS Report RL32909, *Federal Protection for Human Research Subjects: An Analysis of the Common Rule and Its Interactions with FDA Regulations and the HIPAA Privacy Rule*, by Erin D. Williams.

[44] CDRH, FDA, *Humanitarian Device Exemptions Regulation*: Questions and Answers; Final Guidance for Industry, July 12, 2001

[45] A general purpose reagent is "a chemical reagent that has general laboratory application, is used to collect, prepare, and examine specimens from the human body for diagnostic purposes, and is not labeled or otherwise intended for a specific diagnostic application ... [General purpose reagents] do not include laboratory machinery, automated or powered systems" (21 CFR § 864.4010).

[46] Analyte specific reagents (ASRs) are "antibodies, both polyclonal and monoclonal, specific receptor proteins, ligands, nucleic acid sequences, and similar reagents which, through specific binding or chemical reaction with substances in a specimen, are intended for use in a diagnostic application for identification and quantification of an individual chemical substance or ligand in biological specimens" (21 CFR § 864. 4020(a)).

[47] In 2006, FDA's OIVD issued two draft guidance documents on IVDs: "Draft Guidance for Industry and FDA Staff - Commercially Distributed Analyte Specific Reagents (ASRs): Frequently Asked Questions," (September 7, 2006) and "In Vitro Diagnostic Multivariate Index Assays," (September 7, 2007)

[48] FDA, Overview of IVD Regulation, March 4, 2003

[49] See "Find Device CLIA '88 Categorization," *OIVD, FDA website* (December 2005)

[50] "Clinical Laboratory Improvement Amendments (CLIA) Overview," *CMS Website* (December 18, 2006)

[51] United States v. Research Laboratories, Inc., 126 F.2d 42 (9th Cir. 1942).

[52] 21 CFR §§ 801.405 to 801.437. Denture repair kits, impact resistant lenses in sunglasses and eyeglasses, ozone emission levels, chlorofluorocarbon propellants, hearing aids, menstrual tampons, chlorofluorocarbons or other ozone depleting substances, latex condoms, and devices containing natural rubber.

[53] FDA, *Good Manufacturing Practice/Quality Systems*

[54] OIVD, which reviews clinical laboratory test kits and equipment, has the capacity for both premarket scientific review and pre- and postmarket compliance activity.

[55] See ORA

[56] United States House of Representatives Committee on Government Reform Minority Staff, *Prescription for Harm: The Decline in FDA Enforcement Activity*, Special Investigation prepared for Representative Henry A. Waxman (June 2006), p. I

[57] Recall does not include market withdrawal or a stock recovery. A market withdrawal is a firm's removal or correction of a distributed product for a minor violation that does not violate the law and would not be subject to legal action by FDA, e.g., normal stock rotation practices, routine equipment adjustments and repairs, etc. Stock recovery involves correction of a problem before product is shipped (i.e., is still in the manufacturer's control).

[58] CRS Report RL34 167, *The FDA's Authority to Recall Products*, by Vanessa K. Burrows.

[59] For further information about product liability, see CRS Report RL3 3423, *Products Liability: A Legal Overview*, by Henry Cohen and Vanessa K. Burrows.

[60] *Riegel v. Medtronic, Inc.*, 522 U.S. ___ (2008).

[61] *Wyeth v. Levine*, 555 U.S. ___ (2009).

[62] P.L. 110-85, sec. 225.

[63] U.S. Government Accountability Office, *Medical Devices: FDA Should Take Steps to Ensure That High-Risk Device Types Are Approved through the Most Stringent Premarket Review Process*, GAO-09-190, January 2009

[64] There are some pricing restrictions for devices HDE devices. For details, see CRS Report RL34571, *Medical Device User Fees and User Fee Acts*, by Erin D. Williams.

[65] For further information about Medicare, see CRS Report RL33712, *Medicare: A Primer*, by Jennifer O'Sullivan.

[66] For further information, see CRS Report RL33 832, *Genetic Testing: Scientific Background for Policymakers*, by Amanda K. Sarata.

[67] For example, see S. 301.

[68] For further information about the Animal Welfare Act, see CRS Report RS22493, *The Animal Welfare Act: Background and Selected Legislation*, by Geoffrey S. Becker.

[69] For further information about exportation to Cuba and other related issues, see CRS Report RL33819, *Cuba: Issues for the 110th Congress*, by Mark P. Sullivan.

INDEX

A

B

C

D

E

F

G

H

I

J

K

L

M

N

O

P

Q

R

S

T

U